Pre-Obstetric Emergency Training

SECOND EDITION

T0257206

Pre-Obstetric Emergency Training

A Practical Approach

SECOND EDITION

Advanced Life Support Group

EDITED BY

Mark Woolcock

WILEY Blackwell

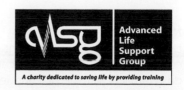

This edition first published 2019 © 2019 by John Wiley & Sons Ltd

Edition History
Wiley-Blackwell (1e, 2009)

All rights reserved. No part of this publication may be reproduced, stored in a retrieval system, or transmitted, in any form or by any means, electronic, mechanical, photocopying, recording or otherwise, except as permitted by law. Advice on how to obtain permission to reuse material from this title is available at http://www.wiley.com/go/permissions.

The right of Advanced Life Support Group (ALSG) to be identified as the authors of the editorial material in this work has been asserted in accordance with law.

Registered Office(s)
John Wiley & Sons, Inc., 111 River Street, Hoboken, NJ 07030, USA
John Wiley & Sons Ltd, The Atrium, Southern Gate, Chichester, West Sussex, PO19 8SQ, UK

Editorial Office
9600 Garsington Road, Oxford, OX4 2DQ, UK

For details of our global editorial offices, customer services, and more information about Wiley products visit us at www.wiley.com.

Wiley also publishes its books in a variety of electronic formats and by print-on-demand. Some content that appears in standard print versions of this book may not be available in other formats.

Limit of Liability/Disclaimer of Warranty
The contents of this work are intended to further general scientific research, understanding, and discussion only and are not intended and should not be relied upon as recommending or promoting scientific method, diagnosis, or treatment by physicians for any particular patient. In view of ongoing research, equipment modifications, changes in governmental regulations, and the constant flow of information relating to the use of medicines, equipment, and devices, the reader is urged to review and evaluate the information provided in the package insert or instructions for each medicine, equipment, or device for, among other things, any changes in the instructions or indication of usage and for added warnings and precautions. While the publisher and authors have used their best efforts in preparing this work, they make no representations or warranties with respect to the accuracy or completeness of the contents of this work and specifically disclaim all warranties, including without limitation any implied warranties of merchantability or fitness for a particular purpose. No warranty may be created or extended by sales representatives, written sales materials or promotional statements for this work. The fact that an organization, website, or product is referred to in this work as a citation and/or potential source of further information does not mean that the publisher and authors endorse the information or services the organization, website, or product may provide or recommendations it may make. This work is sold with the understanding that the publisher is not engaged in rendering professional services. The advice and strategies contained herein may not be suitable for your situation. You should consult with a specialist where appropriate. Further, readers should be aware that websites listed in this work may have changed or disappeared between when this work was written and when it is read. Neither the publisher nor authors shall be liable for any loss of profit or any other commercial damages, including but not limited to special, incidental, consequential, or other damages.

A catalogue record for this book is available from the Library of Congress and the British Library.

9781119348382

Cover images: © ideabug/iStockphoto; Jade and Bertrand Maitre/Getty Images; sturti/Getty Images; Mark Woolcock, NHS Cornwall 111
Cover design by Wiley

Set in 10/12 pt MyriadPro Light by SPi Global, Pondicherry, India

Printed and bound by CPI Group (UK) Ltd, Croydon, CR0 4YY

C9781119348382_270224

Note to text
Drugs and their doses are mentioned in this text. Although every effort has been made to ensure accuracy, the writers, editors, publishers and printers cannot accept liability for errors or omissions. The final responsibility for delivery of the correct dose remains with the practitioner administering the drug.

Contents

Working group

Contributors

Sam Fournier   Paramedic, Educator, Ecole Supérieure d'Ambulancier et Soins d'Urgence Romande, Lausanne, Switzerland

Kim Hinshaw   FRCOG
Consultant Obstetrician and Gynaecologist, Director of Research & Innovation, City Hospitals Sunderland NHS Foundation Trust
Visiting Professor, University of Sunderland

Paul Holmes   MRCOG
Consultant Obstetrician and Gynaecologist, NHS Forth Valley

Denise Mace   MSc Advanced Clinical Practice, BSc(Hons) Midwifery
Delivery Suite Coordinator, City Hospitals Sunderland NHS Foundation Trust

Faye Rodger   FRCOG
Consultant Obstetrician and Gynaecologist, NHS Borders

Fiona Scarlett   BSc (Hons) Healthcare Practice, MCPara
Emergency Practitioner (Paramedic), Surrey and Sussex Healthcare NHS Trust

Helen Simpson   MRCOG
Consultant Obstetrician, South Tees Hospitals NHS Foundation Trust

Martin Smith   FRCEM
Consultant Emergency Medicine, Salford Royal NHS Foundation Trust, Salford

Martin Thomas   MD FRCS(A&E)Ed. MRCP FRCEM
Consultant in Emergency Medicine, Emergency Department, Salford Royal NHS Foundation Trust, Salford

Aarti Ullal   MRCOG
Consultant Obstetrician and Gynaecologist, City Hospitals Sunderland NHS Foundation Trust

Susan Wieteska   CEO, Advanced Life Support Group, Manchester

Mark Woolcock   Consultant Paramedic, Cornwall

Contributors

Contributors to second edition

Sally Buller
Registered Nurse RM Registered Midwife RM
Senior Specialist Midwife/Project lead for Maternity notes, Perinatal Institute

Brigid Hayden
FRCOG
Obstetrician & Gynaecologist, Member of MOET Working Group, Member of POET Working Group

Amanda Mansfield
Consultant Midwife
Medical Directorate, London Ambulance Service

Jonathan Wyllie
FRCPCH FRCP
Professor of Neonatology and Paediatrics, University of Durham
Consultant Neonatologist, Clinical Director of Neonatology, South Tees NHS Foundation Trust
Vice President Resuscitation Council UK

Contributors to first edition

Sally Evans   Midwifery, *Middlesbrough*

Kim Hinshaw   Obstetrics and Gynaecology, *Sunderland*

Helen Simpson   Obstetrics and Gynaecology, *Middlesbrough*

Mark Woolcock   Pre-Hospital Care, *Truro*

Malcolm Woollard   Pre-Hospital Care, *Coventry*

Jonathan Wyllie   Neonatology, *Middlesbrough*

Dedication

With thanks to our families and friends for their tolerance, support and understanding during the review and rewriting of this second edition manual and its associated course.

Foreword to second edition

I am privileged to have been asked to write this introduction to the second edition of the POET manual. Over the last 9 years POET has offered pragmatic advice and skills training to a wide range of practitioners working in the pre-hospital environment. The manual and course encompass the full range of situations found in maternity care, from normal delivery to complex antenatal and intrapartum complications which put both the mother and fetus at risk.

In total more than 1500 professionals have benefited from this training and this has included paramedics, ambulance technicians, midwives, emergency department teams, primary care physicians and others. The first edition of the manual has been translated into Polish (2011) and Japanese (2014) and courses are run regularly in the UK, the Netherlands and Switzerland under the auspices of the Advanced Life Support Group (ALSG), Manchester, UK. The Working Group is also multi-national with members from across the UK and Europe. Experienced faculty now includes ambulance personnel working closely with obstetricians, neonatologists and midwives to deliver high-quality practical training to increase both confidence and skills to the multidisciplinary team in the pre-hospital setting. The dedication of faculty ensures the ongoing success of the course, with many teaching enthusiastically in their own time.

The manual has been comprehensively updated. It now includes a review of the UK maternal mortality reports produced annually by MBRRACE (https://www.npeu.ox.ac.uk/mbrrace-uk) and highlights the importance of non-technical skills (clear communication, decision making and team working) in the area of pre-hospital maternity care. This new edition continues to offer clear and practical advice to all professionals involved in pre-hospital maternity care – congratulations to the wider POET team.

Kim Hinshaw FRCOG
Consultant Obstetrician & Gynaecologist; Director of Research & Innovation
City Hospitals Sunderland NHS Foundation Trust
Visiting Professor
University of Sunderland
2018

Acknowledgements

Many people have worked hard to produce this book and the accompanying course. The editor thanks all the contributors for their efforts and all POET providers and instructors who took the time to send their comments during the reviews of the text and the course, in particular Brigid Hayden who completed a very detailed review of the manual.

We are all greatly indebted to Kate Wieteska for producing the line drawings that illustrate the text, and Kirsten Baxter at ALSG for her support and organisational skills. We thank the ALSG/CAI Emergency Maternal and Child Health (EMCH) programme, the ALSG Managing Obstetric Emergencies and Trauma (MOET) course and the Resuscitation Council for the shared use of some of their line drawings and algorithms. We gratefully acknowledge the written information and guidance received from the Perinatal Institute. Also, we thank the Consultant Midwife Amanda Mansfield from London Ambulance Service and Matthew Davis Clinical Fellow in Primary Care from South Western Ambulance Service for sharing their organisations' photographs.

We would like to thank all of those in advance who attend the POET course and others using this text for their continued constructive comments regarding the future development of both the course and the manual.

Preface to second edition

2009…

Looking back at the preface to the first edition, a clear picture was painted depicting a distinct gap in the paramedic curriculum and the paucity of exposure to bespoke obstetric training and education. The 2009 manual was thus intended to support those working in the pre-hospital arena. The principles were set firmly in the didactic realms of paramedic practice and whilst this assisted those working in the 999 services, it had less appeal to other healthcare professionals working in unscheduled and urgent care settings, and an increasing amount who worked 'in-hospital'.

Some 9 years later, the paradigmatic shift of paramedic education from in-house training schools to academic institutions is producing highly autonomous, degree-educated practitioners who demand detailed, evidence-based texts and materials to underpin focused learning.

Concurrently, the centralisation of obstetric services has placed an increasing requirement on Emergency Department staff to manage patients with obstetric emergencies without any specialised cover. The need has never been greater for a multidisciplinary course that prepares healthcare professionals to promptly recognise and effectively manage a wide range of obstetric emergencies.

Now…

As hinted above, the term 'pre-hospital' in the title of the manual and course suggested a narrow field of practice. The working group has spent many hours debating what the most descriptive title would be, enabling immediate acknowledgement of what and whom this manual is for. It was tremendously difficult to settle on a title that recognises midwives, paramedics, nurses and doctors, who may encounter patients in their own houses, in ambulances or in hospitals without any obstetric services. It was decided that the term 'pre-obstetric emergency training' was most encompassing and would provide guidance for managing patients when no obstetric staff or facilities were available.

The future…

The face of modern healthcare is changing rapidly. In primary care and out-of-hours services, the models are now GP lead as opposed to exclusively GP delivered and the use of advanced nurse and paramedic practitioners is burgeoning. It is expected that within the next 5 years one-third of all registered paramedics will be working outside of ambulance trusts in a range of settings and roles never previously associated with this profession.

The second edition manual, the updated course and powerful e-learning have all been updated and revamped to assist the modern generalist clinician develop confidence when dealing with specialist situations, building a foundation for future safe practice.

Mark Woolcock
2018

Preface to first edition

Pre-hospital obstetric incidents make up a significant proportion of the more costly litigation claims against UK ambulance services. These claims are based either on an alleged failure to identify and manage a problem or lack of appropriate equipment for the treatment of a preterm baby.

For a number of years after the UK national paramedic curriculum was introduced in the UK, it included no specific training on the management of obstetric emergencies at an 'advanced life support' level. Most staff received only a half-day of lectures during their initial ambulance technician training at the beginning of their career. Since 1999, advanced obstetrics and gynaecology became a mandatory part of the paramedic course for new entrants but with the expectation that existing paramedics would receive update training. Our experience has indicated, however, that paramedics in many parts of the UK have not had the opportunity to do so.

A confidential enquiry into maternal and child health (CEMACH) report has indicated that many of the pregnant women dying 'had chaotic lifestyles and found it hard to engage with maternity services'. The ambulance service may be the initial contact with the health service for these patients and their peers who become unwell but are fortunate enough to survive. The CEMACH report identifies the need for a widened awareness of the risk factors and early signs and symptoms of potentially serious problems in pregnancy, and makes a number of key recommendations that could be addressed in part by appropriately trained pre-hospital practitioners. For example, it states:

All clinical staff must undertake regular, written, documented and audited training for:

- The identification, initial management and referral for serious medical and mental health conditions which, although unrelated to pregnancy, may affect pregnant women or recently delivered mothers
- The early recognition and management of severely ill pregnant women and impending maternal collapse
- The improvement of basic, immediate and advanced life support skills. A number of courses provide additional training for staff caring for pregnant women and newborn babies

There is also a need for staff to recognise their limitations and to know when, how and whom to call for assistance.

This manual and its associated Advanced Life Support Group training course (also called POET) hope to meet these educational needs for a range of pre-hospital practitioners. Both the text and the course have been developed by a multi-disciplinary team of senior paramedics, consultant obstetricians and midwives, all of whom are practicing clinicians and experienced educators. POET course teaching teams have a similar multi-professional membership with a shared philosophy of combining pre-hospital and obstetric expertise. Although we anticipate that paramedics and pre-hospital physicians will make up the bulk of our readership and course candidates, POET will also be of value to nurses working in walk-in and unscheduled care centres and to midwives and to GPs – particularly those working at a distance from further support.

It is our sincere hope that POET will build the confidence and competence of pre-hospital practitioners and thus contribute to reducing the incidence of maternal and fetal mortality and morbidity.

Malcolm Woollard
Helen Simpson
Kim Hinshaw
Sue Wieteska
November 2009

Contact details and website information

ALSG: www.alsg.org

For details on ALSG courses visit the website or contact:
Advanced Life Support Group
ALSG Centre for Training and Development
29–31 Ellesmere Street
Swinton, Manchester
M27 0LA
Tel: +44 (0) 161 794 1999
Fax: +44 (0) 161 794 9111
Email: enquiries@alsg.org

Updates

The material contained within this book is updated on approximately a four-yearly cycle. However, practice may change in the interim period. We will post any changes on the ALSG website, so we advise you to visit the website regularly to check for updates (www.alsg.org/uk/poet).

References

To access references visit the ALSG website www.alsg.org – references are on the course pages. To access country-specific Legal and Ethical Issues for POET, visit the ALSG website www.alsg.org/legal.

On-line feedback

It is important to ALSG that the contact with our providers continues after a course is completed. We now contact everyone 6 months after his or her course has taken place asking for on-line feedback on the course. This information is then used whenever the course is updated to ensure that the course provides optimum training to its participants.

How to use your textbook

The anytime, anywhere textbook

Wiley E-Text

Your textbook comes with free access to a **Wiley E-Text: Powered by VitalSource** version – a digital, interactive version of this textbook which you own as soon as you download it.

Your **Wiley E-Text** allows you to:

Search: Save time by finding terms and topics instantly in your book, your notes, even your whole library (once you've downloaded more textbooks)

Note and Highlight: Colour code, highlight and make digital notes right in the text so you can find them quickly and easily

Organize: Keep books, notes and class materials organized in folders inside the application

Share: Exchange notes and highlights with friends, classmates and study groups

Upgrade: Your textbook can be transferred when you need to change or upgrade computers

Link: Link directly from the page of your interactive textbook to all of the material contained on the companion website

The **Wiley E-Text** version will also allow you to copy and paste any photograph or illustration into assignments, presentations and your own notes.

To access your Wiley E-Text:

- Visit **http://support.wiley.com** to request a redemption code via the 'Live Chat' or 'Ask A Question' tabs (with a proof of purchase).
- Go to **https://online.vitalsource.co.uk** and log in or create an account. Go to Redeem and enter your redemption code to add this book to your library.
- Or to download the Bookshelf application to your computer, tablet or mobile device go to **www.vitalsource.com/software/bookshelf/downloads**.
- Open the Bookshelf application on your computer and register for an account.
- Follow the registration process and enter your redemption code to download your digital book.

The VitalSource Bookshelf can now be used to view your Wiley E-Text on iOS, Android and Kindle Fire!

- **For iOS:** Visit the app store to download the VitalSource Bookshelf: **http://bit.ly/17ib3XS**
- **For Android and Kindle Fire:** Visit the Google Play Market to download the VitalSource Bookshelf: **http://bit.ly/BSAAGP**

You can now sign in with the email address and password you used when you created your VitalSource Bookshelf Account.

Full E-Text support for mobile devices is available at: **http://support.vitalsource.com**

We hope you enjoy using your new textbook. Good luck with your studies!

CHAPTER 1
Obstetric services

Learning outcomes

After reading this chapter, you will be able to:
- Discuss the relationship between the different professional groups involved in the management of the obstetric patient
- Describe the function and importance of hand-held records and how to use them effectively

1.1 Organisation of obstetric services, epidemiology of obstetric emergencies and role of the ambulance service, general practitioner and midwife

Organisation

Around 700 000 women a year use obstetric services. The birth rate in the United Kingdom (UK) has slowed in recent years following a rise throughout the last decade. Multidisciplinary teams provide maternity services with midwifery and obstetric medical staff working together to provide optimal care. Community midwives perform the majority of care in the out-of-hospital setting. Inpatient antenatal care is now uncommon and not usually for long periods. Similarly, the postnatal length of stay for all women, including those delivered by caesarean section, has been reduced with the majority of care occurring in the community.

General practitioners (GPs) have in recent years become less and less involved in all aspects of pregnancy care, although there are still a small number who are involved in care in labour.

Place of delivery

The *Maternity Matters* report confirmed that women should be the central focus of obstetric care, emphasising the need for those providing obstetric services to support women in making informed choices and to provide easy access to care (DoH, 2007). Women undergo a risk assessment prior to delivery to help them choose where to deliver. This assessment is undertaken by their midwife in conjunction with medical staff, if required, and will involve assessment of previous medical history, previous obstetric history and the progress of the current pregnancy. The women will then be offered advice to help them choose the place of birth.

A woman may choose to have a home birth; deliver in a midwife-led unit, which may be either 'stand-alone' or attached to a consultant-led unit (co-located); or deliver in a consultant-led unit. Women may also choose to 'free birth': a growing phenomenon in which the baby is delivered unassisted and unattended by a healthcare professional. Whilst this is perfectly legal, one should note it is illegal for someone without midwifery qualifications to assist in the birth unless in an emergency.

The 2011 Birthplace in England study identified that nulliparous women (those having their first baby) were more at risk for adverse perinatal outcomes (stillbirth, neonatal encephalopathy, brachial plexus injury, clavicle fracture, etc.) with a planned

Pre-Obstetric Emergency Training: A Practical Approach, Second Edition. Edited by Mark Woolcock.
© 2019 John Wiley & Sons Ltd. Published 2019 by John Wiley & Sons Ltd.

home birth than multiparous women (BECG, 2011). There was no statistical increase in risk for adverse outcomes for nulliparous women delivering in a midwife-led unit. It was found that for multiparous women, there is no increased risk for adverse outcomes between each planned place of delivery. It was also found that women who plan to deliver at home or in a midwife-led unit are more likely to have a 'natural' birth with reduced interventions compared with those who deliver in an obstetric unit. Choosing an appropriate place of delivery relies on effective communication between healthcare professionals and women regarding any specific risk factors.

In the majority of cases, women choose the appropriate place to deliver their baby. Midwives have a duty of care to support the woman's final choice of place for delivery even if there are factors that make this a high-risk decision. Occasionally this causes difficulties, for example, in home delivery where access is poor, there is no phone signal or the home environment is less than ideal. Some women with a high-risk pregnancy also request home delivery. As long as the woman has capacity (see Chapter 2), is informed of the risks to herself and her baby and is not under duress, she is entitled to make that decision.

Mode of delivery

The majority of deliveries are uncomplicated, however the national caesarean section rate is 26.2% of births. In contrast, the rate in 1990 was only 12%. Caesarean section delivery requires major surgery and can have significant associated risks for both mother and baby.

Common pre-hospital emergencies

- Labour +/− delivery (term or preterm)
- Bleeding antenatally or postnatally (including miscarriage) and postoperative vaginal haemorrhage
- Abdominal pain other than labour
- Pre-eclampsia and eclampsia (this is now less common: 2:10 000 cases due to the use of magnesium sulphate in hospital in at-risk cases; however, this does mean that one of the more common places to have a convulsion will be in the community)
- Prolapsed umbilical cord

Transfer

Transfer may be necessary where risk factors develop before or during labour and after birth that necessitate moving the woman or baby from one location to another. Transfer may be required from all places of delivery.

In the 2011 Birthplace in England study, it was found that for the three non-obstetric unit settings (home, stand-alone midwifery unit and co-located midwifery unit), transfer rates were much higher for nulliparous women (36–45%) than for multiparous women (9–13%).

Common reasons for transfer from home or from a midwife-led unit are concerns about the progress of labour, fetal or maternal well-being, or neonatal well-being. A common reason for transfer between consultant-led obstetric units is the need to access a neonatal cot for the baby either because the unit they are in does not have the appropriate neonatal facilities or all the cots are full. In these situations, the outcome is better for the baby if they are transferred while still in utero rather than after delivery. Occasionally, women need to be moved to other units for maternal specialist care.

Generally, a midwife (or medical staff) will accompany the woman and will be an invaluable source of advice and knowledge if problems occur during transfer. See Table 1.1 for the roles undertaken by clinical staff.

Further information on the management of inter-hospital transfers generally and neonatal transfers specifically can be found in the Neonatal Adult Paediatric Safe Transfer and Retrieval (NAPSTaR) manual (Fortune et al., 2019).

TOP TIP

Many features of the clinical management of an obstetric patient during secondary transfer are similar to that required in the home or during primary hospital admission. For example, remember to transport the patient who is unable to maintain their own position in the 15–30° left lateral tilt position or manually displace the uterus.

Table 1.1 Roles of healthcare staff

	Paramedic	Midwife	GP (if on scene)	Obstetrician (via telephone)
Clinical condition	Assess	Assess	Assess	
Initiate holding treatment	Advanced life support (ALS) Obstetric support	Assist with ALS Obstetric expertise	Assist with ALS Obstetric support*	Advise on treatment
Transfer	Provide transportation Liaise with receiving unit Confirm exact location of receiving obstetric unit within hospital	Advise on most appropriate receiving unit Liaise with receiving unit Advise on timing/ need for transfer		Advise on most appropriate receiving unit Liaise with referring crew Advise on timing/need for transfer
Advice	Transportation options/ positioning in the ambulance	Obstetric expertise	General issues	Obstetric expertise

*Some GPs have specific expertise in obstetrics.

Admissions procedures

These depend on local policies. Obstetric patients are usually admitted directly to the obstetric service via a triage assessment unit or delivery suite. In the case of major trauma, obstetric patients should be transferred to the emergency department or major trauma centre depending on the systems in place locally. In the case of medical problems admit via urgent care pathways.

In many units, women with problems in early pregnancy will be admitted to the gynaecology department via an early pregnancy assessment unit.

1.2 Using patient hand-held notes

Most maternity units in the UK provide women with their own maternity hand-held notes. Figure 1.1 shows an example of the national pregnancy notes that are currently used by approximately 60% of obstetric units in England (produced by the Perinatal Institute www.preg.info; accessed February 2018).

The pregnancy notes aim to facilitate a partnership between the mother, her family and the care provider, placing emphasis on patient safety and informed choice. They are designed to 'support comprehensive history taking, promote effective communication between the mother and the multidisciplinary care team and between members of that team'. The notes are given to the woman by her midwife at her booking appointment in early pregnancy, enabling the expectant mother and her family to be informed and involved in decisions that affect her and her baby. To deal with special issues during pregnancy, a personalised management plan will outline specific outline specific treatment and care agreed between the mother and her care team. This plan will be reviewed at each antenatal contact and updated if the mother's risks/needs change.

The woman's medical/obstetric and social details are available to all healthcare professionals who may care for her during her pregnancy.

The notes enable effective communication within the multidisciplinary team, including ambulance clinicians who may attend the woman in her home or the community. All clinicians should document clinical care in these notes when they attend a woman during pregnancy if she is not transferred. Contemporaneous record keeping is a fundamental component of good clinical practice. Therefore the hand-held pregnancy notes are an important link for healthcare professionals to improve care and reduce error.

NHS No. | Maternity Unit |

CONFIDENTIAL

These notes should be carried by the expectant mother at all times during her pregnancy. If found, please return the notes immediately to the owner, or her midwife or maternity unit.

NHS

Pregnancy

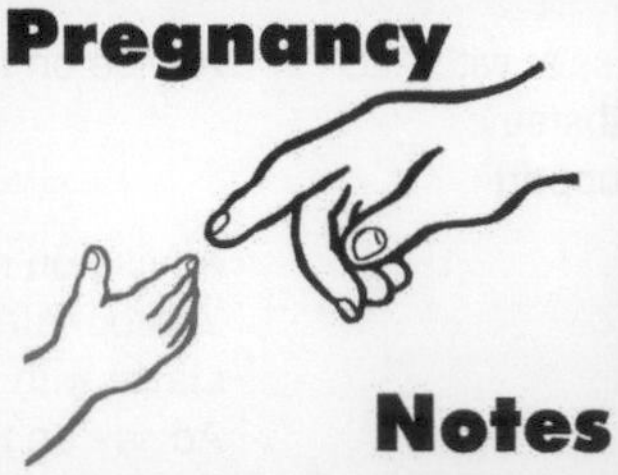

Notes

First name | Surname

Address

Postcode | ☎

Date of birth | D D M M Y Y | Unit No.

These Pregnancy Notes are a guide to your options during pregnancy, and are intended to help you make informed choices. The explanations in these notes are a general guide only, and not everything will be relevant to you. If you are asked to make a choice, feel free to ask any questions. Talk about your options with family/friends, write down anything you want to discuss and take it to your appointment. Key questions are:- What are my options? What are the advantages/disadvantages for each option for me? How do I get support to help me make a decision that is right for me? Additional information will also be available in leaflets which you will be given as needed.

EDD | D D M M Y Y

Communication

Assistance required No☐ Yes☐ Details | Your preferred name

Do you speak English No☐ Yes☐ What is your first language

Preferred language | Interpreter ☎

Plan of care

Depending on your circumstances, you and your partner will have the choice between midwifery based care or maternity team based care during your pregnancy. Please discuss your choices/options with your midwife. This will be based on your individual medical and obstetric history.

Date recorded	Planned place of birth	Lead professional	Job title	Reason if changed
D D M M Y Y				
D D M M Y Y				
D D M M Y Y				

Maternity contacts

Named Midwife | ☎

Maternity Unit | ☎

Antenatal Clinic ☎ | Delivery Suite ☎

Community Office ☎ | Ambulance ☎

Primary care contacts

Centre | ☎ | Other(s)

GP | Initial | Surname | ☎

Postcode (GP) | ☎

Health Visitor | ☎

Next of Kin

Name

Address

☎ | Relation

Emergency Contact

Name

Address

☎ | ☎

NHS Information Service for Parents
Sign up for emails and texts at www.nhs.uk/parents

page 1

Figure 1.1 Example of national patient hand-held records. (Reproduced with kind permission of the Perinatal Institute)

Plans for Pregnancy and Parenthood

Topics	Discussed	Signature* and Date	Your intentions or preferences	Leaflets given
Preparing for your new baby		D D M M Y Y		
Parent education	☐			☐
Hospital visit	☐			
Safe sleeping	☐			
Home environment	☐			
Equipment	☐			
Newborn screening and examination	☐			
Vitamin K	☐			☐
BCG (see p26)		D D M M Y Y		
Baby BCG indicated No ☐ Yes ☐			Reason:	
Discussed with mother No ☐ Yes ☐ N/A ☐				
Mother agrees to vaccine No ☐ Yes ☐			If no, reason declined	
Leaflet: 'TB, BCG vaccine and your baby' given to mother No ☐ Yes ☐ N/A ☐				
Connecting with your baby		D D M M Y Y		☐
Talking to your baby	☐			
Noticing and responding to baby's movements	☐			
How this can help your baby's brain development	☐			
Greeting your baby for the first time		D D M M Y Y		☐
Skin to skin contact	☐			
Keeping baby close	☐			
Recognising feeding cues	☐			
Responding to your baby's needs		D D M M Y Y		☐
Importance of comfort and love to help baby's brain develop	☐			
Responsive feeding	☐			
Feeding your baby		D D M M Y Y		☐
Value of breastfeeding as protection, comfort and food	☐			
Getting off to a good start	☐			
Understanding how a baby breastfeeds	☐			
Where to get help including local support groups	☐			

Confirmation that a conversation has taken place around the topics outlined above

Comments	Signature & date

* Signatures must be listed on page 30 for identification

Name

Unit No/ NHS No

page 27

Figure 1.1 (*Continued*)

Although there is variation in maternity hand-held notes throughout the UK, the same general principles apply throughout:

- The front cover will display the woman's name, address, named midwife, consultant and GP, next of kin and emergency contact
- Information within the notes for the woman to read, including appropriate support groups/advice line numbers, screening tests, pregnancy complications and routine visits
- The notes will identify whether the woman is on the low- or high-risk pathway of care. This is dependent on factors identified at the beginning of the pregnancy. The pathway may change during the pregnancy if complications arise, e.g. gestational diabetes, pre-eclampsia, obstetric cholestasis
- The antenatal section will display all screening tests/investigations performed, routine antenatal visits, scan results and fetal growth monitoring
- There will be a section for the woman to complete a birth plan, in discussion with her midwife
- There is a labour and postnatal section, which also includes detailed information regarding the baby, such as condition at birth, findings on the neonatal examination and details on feeding
- **Most hand-held notes have an alert/special features section**. This will identify any complications or potential complications, and may show a plan of care to address these complications. A plan of care could also be documented in the management plan section. **Any healthcare professional can and should annotate this page**
- There will be a section for correspondence between healthcare professionals, identifying potential problems and formulating plans of care. **Any healthcare professional can and should annotate this page**
- Ambulance clinicians attending an obstetric patient who has not been transported to hospital should leave a copy of their patient report form in the hand-held records. If a written or printed copy cannot be left, the hand-held notes must be annotated

It is paramount that the hand-held notes accompany the woman for all hospital admissions and routine antenatal visits. However, the notes may not have been issued to a woman in very early pregnancy if she has not booked through her midwife.

Summary of key points

- It is important that you are aware of the roles of other healthcare professionals in the care of the obstetric patient
- Remember that any health professional can and should annotate the alert page in the patient's hand-held notes

CHAPTER 2
Legal and ethical issues

Learning outcomes

After reading this chapter, you will be able to:
- Discuss the impact of obstetric-related incidents on litigation claims
- Describe the principles of gaining consent from adult patients and minors
- Discuss the principles of maintaining patient confidentiality and the legal context
- Debate the appropriateness of recognising death in obstetric cases
- State the common causes of complaints
- Define clinical negligence and describe the components necessary to demonstrate its proof
- Discuss the impact of varied cultural issues on the provision of obstetric care in the pre-hospital setting
- State the professional responsibilities of pre-hospital practitioners

---

This chapter outlines the principles involved in law and ethics. The specifics of legal and other frameworks for specific countries is available on-line (www.alsg.org/uk/le).

2.1 Impact of litigation claims

The NHS Litigation Authority (NHSLA) report *Ten Years of Maternity Claims* (NHSLA, 2012) identified that maternity claims were the second largest group of claims and accounted for the highest value (49%) of the total value of claims under the Clinical Negligence Scheme for Trusts (CNST). A significant proportion of the more costly litigation claims made against UK ambulance services arise from pre-hospital obstetric incidents. Although in a 10-year period, obstetric cases consisted of only 13 of the total 272 claims, the average value of these cases was £815 000. Four were valued at more than £1 million. Claims were based on either an alleged failure to identify and manage a problem or a lack of appropriate equipment for the treatment of a preterm baby. The largest claim was for £3 375 000 and related to an alleged lack of equipment to care for a baby born at 26 weeks (Dobbie and Cooke, 2008).

Although the numbers of women and babies dying as a result of obstetric emergencies in the UK are small, some of these deaths might be prevented if effective training in the prompt recognition and management of these cases is undertaken by pre-hospital providers (Woollard et al., 2008). Although it could be argued that antenatal provision of preventative obstetric care is more effective than treating problems after they arise, the Confidential Enquiry into Maternal and Child Health (CEMACH) report of 2007 suggested that many of the pregnant women who died 'had chaotic lifestyles and found it hard to engage with maternity services' (CEMACH, 2007a). One of its 'top ten' recommendations stated:

All clinical staff must undertake regular, written, documented and audited training for the

- Identification, initial management and referral for serious medical and mental health conditions which, although unrelated to pregnancy, may affect pregnant women or recently delivered mothers

---

Pre-Obstetric Emergency Training: A Practical Approach, Second Edition. Edited by Mark Woolcock.
© 2019 John Wiley & Sons Ltd. Published 2019 by John Wiley & Sons Ltd.

- Early recognition and management of severely ill pregnant women and impending maternal collapse
- Improvement of basic, immediate and advanced life support skills. A number of courses provide additional training for staff caring for pregnant women and newborn babies

There is also a need for staff to recognise their limitations and to know when, how and whom to call for assistance (CEMACH, 2007a).

All registered healthcare professionals are ultimately responsible for identifying and achieving their own training needs and maintaining their own competence. This extends into post-registration training and particularly through continuing professional development activity. A strong motivation for doing so, other than the obvious one of being able to meet patients' needs, is individual accountability for practice. A failure to provide acceptable standards of care not only risks the patient's welfare but also challenges the practitioner's fitness to practice and their right to maintain professional registration. Although obstetric emergencies are rare, the consequences of mishandling them can be particularly severe for mother and baby, as well as for the pre-hospital practitioner.

2.2 Consent and capacity

Healthcare professionals should understand the legal framework within their field of practice, including:

- The legal rights of the mother
- The legal rights of the fetus
- The legal rights of the child
- Consent prior to providing treatment: in particular informed consent and the capacity of the patient to give this. Check the legal framework in your organisation for details of express, implied or presumed consent and ensure that you fulfil the requirements with regard to obtaining this and documenting it

There are often specific caveats in the legal framework where patients are unable to consent and their situation is life threatening. It is important that you understand how this works in your domain.

Capacity and competence of mothers who are minors is a further area that should be well understood by practitioners.

TOP TIP

For consent to be valid the following must pertain:

- **Consent must be given voluntarily**
- **There should be no duress**
- **The patient must have capacity**
- **Any information regarding risks, benefits, side effects and alternatives must be presented in order that the patient can make an informed decision**
- **The patient must be able to communicate their choice**

When obtaining consent from women in labour, take care if they are in pain or under the influence of narcotic analgesics (RCOG, 2015a).

TOP TIP

Remember – patients are allowed to withdraw consent to treatment at any time.

2.3 Confidentiality

All healthcare practitioners have both a professional and a legal duty of confidentiality to their patients.

Guidance and frameworks are produced by relevant professional bodies, employers and data protection legislation.

These apply to all forms of records, not just those stored on computer media.

Consider confidentiality when providing a handover in the emergency department or obstetric unit – never verbally present such information in the presence of relatives or anyone else without the patient's consent. Be particularly vigilant when passing information to colleagues via telephone or radio in the pre-hospital setting.

TOP TIP

When considering confidentiality, you should:

- **Take all reasonable steps to keep a patient's information safe**
- **Obtain the patient's informed consent if you are passing on their information**
- **Only disclose identifiable information if it is absolutely necessary, and, when it is necessary, only disclose the minimum amount necessary**
- **Tell patients when you have disclosed their information**

(Adapted from HCPC, 2012.)

2.4 Recognition of death

The recognition of death is an integral part of healthcare professional practice. Usually, the 'recognition of life extinct' or 'confirmation of death' status is applied when a patient meets the criteria for not attempting cardiopulmonary resuscitation or where attempts at cardiopulmonary resuscitation have failed. Additionally, an advanced decision to refuse treatment or a decision to withdraw life-sustaining treatment may also have been made.

The main aim of perimortem caesarean section (also known as resuscitative hysterotomy) is to increase the woman's cardiac output, thereby improving her chances of survival. Delivery of a live infant may, or may not, also occur. Similarly, in the absence of gross deformities incompatible with life, practitioners should initiate and continue resuscitation attempts for babies that have no signs of life after delivery until handover to emergency department staff.

2.5 Medical errors and negligence

All serious untoward events or *potential* serious untoward events ('near misses') should be reported in accordance with the employer's policy for incident reporting. This ensures that lessons can be learned from mistakes and changes made to training, policy or systems to avoid them being repeated.

Measures are often in place to facilitate lessons learned at the local level being applied on a national scale and this forms an important part of quality control in health services.

All healthcare practitioners are regularly required to deal with situations or people that they consider unpleasant or difficult. If a practitioner inadvertently offends someone, they should use the highly effective strategy of apologising. However, practitioners should not admit to making a clinical error without first taking further advice.

In the event of a complaint being received, practitioners should know the local and national standards set up to handle them, and in particular the time scale within which a response should be provided. They should also understand the appeals process that should be made available to the complainant should they be unhappy with the response.

As has been implied previously, pre-hospital practitioners are accountable for their clinical acts, as well as any clinical omissions. A negligent practitioner is one who has:

> Failed to exercise that degree of care which a person of ordinary prudence with the same or similar training would exercise in the same or similar circumstances. (Woollard and Todd, 2006)

The case of *Bolam v. Friern Hospital Management Committee* (1957) established the precedent that to avoid being considered negligent, a practitioner should provide care to 'the standard of an ordinary man professing to have that special skill …'.

2.6 Cultural issues

Pre-hospital healthcare providers should consider themselves as guests in their patients' homes (or lives). As such they should respect the cultural values of the patients they are asked to attend. They should not expect patients to adhere to other people's personal values.

In many communities it is not normal or acceptable for women to be examined by men, and this can be particularly difficult for patients in the context of gynaecological and obstetric emergencies. Wherever possible, female practitioners should be available to care for such patients and circumstances may require that male providers are not present when intimate examinations or procedures take place. If male practitioners are tempted to take offence in such situations, they should remember that patients have the right of autonomy and self-determination and if such a compromise is necessary to obtain consent to treatment this is well within the patient's rights. If no female practitioners are readily available in an emergency situation, male practitioners should explain the procedures that need to be carried out, and the consequences of delaying them, but ultimately a competent patient has the right to decline them.

2.7 Professional accountability

Registered healthcare practitioners are personally accountable to their registrant body for the care that they provide to patients and have a number of responsibilities set out in their respective codes of conduct. These are similar across professional groups, but the following list is taken from the Health and Care Professions Council's *Standards of Conduct, Performance and Ethics* (HCPC, 2016):

1. You must promote and protect the interests of service users and carers
2. You must communicate appropriately and effectively
3. You must work within the limits of your knowledge
4. You must delegate appropriately
5. You must respect confidentiality
6. You must manage risk
7. You must report concerns about safety
8. You must be open when things go wrong
9. You must be honest and trustworthy
10. You must keep records of your work

2.8 Documentation

A continual thread through this chapter – as well as in following chapters – reminds the practitioner of the importance of accurate and robust clinical documentation. After any patient consultation, which may be either face-to-face, over the telephone or even when providing advice to a colleague, a record should be made either in writing or electronically in the patient's notes. This includes the ambulance patient care record (electronic or paper), the out-of-hours GP record or the patient's hand-held notes.

If the patient is not hospitalised, their patient record should be updated and, where possible, a copy of any written or printed notes included. If a patient is transferred to hospital it is entirely acceptable to complete the patient record after the handover, particularly when managing a clinically unstable patient.

The most important factor is not when the notes were written, but what was recorded. Always strive to maintain the highest level of clinical documentation, as this supports safe and effective patient care. This is not only a requirement of professional registration, but it may also help in your defence against a complaint or allegation of poor practice.

MBRRACE-UK provided a 'very strong recommendation' to ambulance services around patient positioning during transfer with respect to relieving aortocaval compression, and specifically the need to document the woman's position and whether any tilt was used during the journey (MBRRACE-UK, 2014). See Chapter 3.

> **TOP TIP**
>
> **Clinical documentation should:**
>
> - **Be written in a clear, accurate and legible manner**
> - **Record whether consent was obtained or not**
> - **Detail all clinical findings, decisions made and actions taken**
> - **Record the information given to patients**
> - **Record any drugs prescribed or other investigation or treatment**
> - **Identify whether confidential information has been shared**
> - **Always contain details of who is making the record and when**

Summary of key points

- One of the most common subjects of high-cost litigation cases against UK ambulance services is obstetric care
- The Confidential Enquiry into Maternal and Child Health has recommended that all practitioners with a responsibility for caring for obstetric patients receive training in the identification and management of obstetric emergencies
- Informed consent must be sought from all competent adult patients before providing any treatment
- Practitioners have both a professional and legal duty to maintain patient confidentiality and only to use patient data for the purpose for which it was originally collated
- In most circumstances, a pregnant woman should not be pronounced dead in the pre-hospital setting: resuscitation should be initiated and maintained even if the mother has no chance of survival as rarely the fetus may do so
- A non-judgemental and friendly attitude to all patients and an appropriate apology, if needed, will prevent most complaints being made
- Negligence is the failure to act in accordance with the standards of an ordinary person with the same specialist skills
- All registered health practitioners are individually accountable for their own practice
- A high standard of clinical documentation supports safe patient care and also provides a good foundation should any clinical complaint be made

CHAPTER 3

When things go wrong – a review of the MBRRACE-UK and Ireland Maternity Mortality Reports 2014–17

Learning outcomes

After reading this chapter, you will be able to:

- Describe the role of MBRRACE-UK and the background to the confidential enquiries into maternal death in the UK and Ireland
- State the causes of pregnancy-related death, particularly those relating to pre-hospital care practice
- Recognise that *indirect causes* are the main contributor to maternal mortality
- Provide rapid assessment and intervention of pregnancy emergencies at the scene
- Consider which facility is most appropriate for transfer to, ensuring appropriate medical staffing and resource will be available
- Recognise the importance of clear communication with the woman and her family and all practitioners involved in the care of the pregnancy-related emergency
- Recognise that late pregnancy-related deaths (>42 days after the birth) are associated with long-term medical and psychiatric morbidities in women with often complex social lives
- Identify the MBRRACE-UK website as a source of regular updates relevant to pre-hospital care

---

3.1 Introduction

In the UK, maternal mortality in the triennium 2013–15 was reported as 8.8 per 100 000 maternities per year. This was slightly up from the 8.5 per 100 000 reported in the previous report. However, these low figures should not give rise to complacency as the death of any woman related to her pregnancy has significant implications for both her family and society. This chapter will focus particularly (but not exclusively) on the 'lessons learned' that are relevant to pre-hospital care including trauma, and will refer to findings from the enquiries of earlier years. The detailed reports can be found by exploring the MBRRACE-UK (**M**others and **B**abies – **R**educing **R**isk through **A**udit and **C**onfidential **E**nquiries across the **UK**) home page – https://www.npeu.ox.ac.uk/mbrrace-uk (accessed February 2018).

Pre-Obstetric Emergency Training: A Practical Approach, Second Edition. Edited by Mark Woolcock.
© 2019 John Wiley & Sons Ltd. Published 2019 by John Wiley & Sons Ltd.

From a global perspective, it is important to remember that maternal deaths in resource-poor countries are astronomically high, with Sierra Leone in West Africa having the highest estimated maternal death rate of 1.36% (or 1360 per 100 000 maternities per year) – see World Bank data reports at http://data.worldbank.org/indicator/SH.STA.MMRT (accessed February 2018).

3.2 Background

The UK Confidential Enquiry into Maternal Deaths (CEMD) has represented the global gold standard for investigation and improvement in maternity care since its inception in 1952. Rigorous investigation of every case of maternal death during and after pregnancy has highlighted where care can be improved. This is vitally important information for staff, health services and for the family and friends left behind. The CEMD published reports triennially from 1957 until 2008. Similar systems began in Northern Ireland in 1956 and in Scotland in 1965. A UK report has been produced since 1985.

The reports were administered through the Confidential Enquiry into Maternal and Child Health (CEMACH) in 2003 and, from 2009, the Centre for Maternal and Child Health (CMACH). Since 2012, the enquiries have been part of the MBRRACE-UK programme, based at the National Perinatal Epidemiology Unit (NPEU) in Oxford and the enquiries have included data from the Republic of Ireland since then. From 2014, MBRRACE-UK has published an annual report each December, and these contain *topic-specific reviews* of particular interest or concern. Relevant findings will be summarised in subsequent sections. Every reported maternal death is thoroughly scrutinised by an expert panel. There are over 100 independent assessors from many disciplines including emergency medicine. The assessors comment on the 'quality of care' in each case, aligning their assessments to any available evidence-based guidance. The following categories are used:

- Good care; no improvements identified
- Improvements in care identified which would have made no difference to the outcome
- Improvements in care identified which may have made a difference to the outcome

The 'improvements' identified mainly involve care offered by various professional groups or teams, but can include instances where the actions of the woman or her family may have been contributory. The confidential enquiries aim to enhance safety by improving the care offered to women in the UK and Ireland, both during and after pregnancy.

Definitions of maternal death

The World Health Organisation (WHO) uses the following international definitions:

Maternal death	Death of a woman during or up to 6 weeks (42 days) after the end of pregnancy (whether the pregnancy ends by termination, miscarriage, ectopic or birth) through causes associated with, or exacerbated by, pregnancy.
Direct deaths	Deaths resulting from obstetric complications of the pregnant state (pregnancy, labour and the puerperium (i.e. the 6 weeks following delivery)), from interventions, omissions, incorrect treatment or from a chain of events resulting from any of the above (e.g. pre-eclampsia, eclampsia, post-partum haemorrhage, etc.).
Indirect deaths	Deaths resulting from previous existing disease, or disease that developed during pregnancy and which was not the result of direct obstetric causes, but which was aggravated by the physiological effects of pregnancy (e.g. medical and psychiatric disease). (Note: WHO revised the guidance and, from 2016, 'suicide' is reported as a direct cause of maternal death.)
Late deaths	Deaths occurring between 42 days and 1 year after the end of pregnancy that are the result of direct or indirect maternal causes.
Coincidental	Deaths from unrelated causes which happen to occur in pregnancy or the puerperium (e.g. road traffic accidents, homicide, etc.).

Table 3.1 shows the rate of maternal deaths per triennium from 2009 to 2014. There has been a continuing statistically significant reduction in maternal mortality since 2003.

The following summaries are based on the four published MBRRACE-UK reports from 2014 to 2017. General and topic-specific 'key messages' relevant to pre-hospital care practitioners are presented. The topic-specific reviews will continue on a 3-year rolling cycle and the summary reports below include information from the first completed cycle of topic-specific reviews undertaken by MBRRACE-UK.

Table 3.1 Summary of maternal mortality statistics, 2009 to 2014

Triennium	Maternal deaths – direct and indirect (up to 42 days)	Maternities, n	Maternal mortality rate, per 100 000 maternities	Additional coincidental deaths (up to 42 days), n (and rate per 100 000 maternities)
2009–11	253	2 379 014	10.63	23 (0.98)
2010–12	243	2 401 624	10.12	26 (1.08)
2011–13	214	2 373 213	9.02	26 (1.10)
2012–14	200	2 341 745	8.54	41* (1.75)
2013–15	202	2 305 920	8.76	38 (1.65)

*Includes nine deaths due to homicide.

3.3 MBRRACE-UK report 2014 – highlights and take-home messages

Overview

1. Title of report: *Saving Lives, Improving Mothers' Care – Lessons learned to inform future maternity care from the UK and Ireland Confidential Enquiries into Maternal Deaths and Morbidity 2009–2012.*
2. This was the first report to include data for the Republic of Ireland as well as confidential enquiries into the care of women with *severe complications in pregnancy who survived*, with the aim of improving care yet further.
3. Topic-specific reviews included: deaths and morbidity due to sepsis, deaths from haemorrhage, amniotic fluid embolism, anaesthetic-related causes, and neurological and other indirect causes.

Key facts and figures

- The maternal mortality (MM) rate fell to ten per 100 000 maternities, a statistically significant fall of 27% from 2003–05 – (relative risk (RR) 0.73, 95% confidence interval (CI) 0.61–0.86). This fall was mainly due to a 48% fall in *direct* (pregnancy-related) deaths (pre-eclampsia, etc.) (RR 0.52, 95% CI 0.39–0.69).
- Overall, 68% of women died from *indirect* causes, and 32% from *direct* (i.e. pregnancy-related) causes. There was no significant decline in *indirect* (medical and psychiatric) deaths (RR 0.90, 95% CI 0.72–1.11).
- The MM rate from genital tract sepsis *more than halved* from 2006–08 to 2010–12 (RR 0.44, 95% CI 0.22–0.87), but still *almost a quarter of deaths* during pregnancy or up to 42 days after birth were due to sepsis – from influenza and respiratory and urinary infections (one in 11 deaths were due to H1N1 influenza).
- Venous thromboembolism (VTE) was the leading cause of *direct* death and the MM rate from hypertensive disease was the lowest ever recorded.

Key messages – general

- 13% of women who died delivered in an emergency department or an ambulance and 3% delivered at home.
- Two-thirds of women died from *indirect* causes and almost three-quarters of all women who died had coexisting medical complications:
  - Influenza and other non-genital causes of sepsis were the main causes of *indirect* deaths, resulting in a recommendation that influenza vaccination should be actively encouraged.
  - Cardiac, neurological and psychiatric deaths were the next most common indirect causes.
  - 17% had mental health problems, 15% were asthmatic, 22% were overweight and 27% were obese.

> **TOP TIP**
>
> **Pre-hospital care practitioners must be aware of the significant contribution of sepsis and cardiac, neurological and psychiatric disease to maternal death.**

- A recurring theme was that observations were not taken or not responded to. Recommendation – 'All women with any symptoms or signs of ill health, including those who are postnatal, should have a full set of basic observations taken (temperature, pulse rate, respiratory rate and blood pressure), and the results documented and acted on.'

Topic-specific key messages – relevant to pre-hospital care

- *Sepsis* – timely recognition and 'Think Sepsis'. Initiate a sepsis care bundle including prompt administration of intravenous antibiotics.
- *Haemorrhage* – acute point of care estimation of haemoglobin can be falsely reassuring. Fluid resuscitation should be implemented when there is evidence of significant blood loss.
- *Amniotic fluid embolism* – in hospital, peri-mortem caesarean section (PMCS/RH) should be considered if cardiopulmonary resuscitation (CPR) does not restore circulation within 4 minutes. Delays in decision making in hospital were highlighted in the report. In cases of cardiac arrest in the pre-hospital setting, the woman should be transported urgently to the nearest emergency department after initial stabilisation and CPR, where PMCS can be considered. PMCS in the pre-hospital setting will rarely be appropriate.
- *Neurological and other indirect causes* – maternal deaths from *epilepsy* were higher than deaths from hypertensive disorders of pregnancy and many had not received any pre-pregnancy advice. Women with *subarachnoid haemorrhage* (SAH) were not always examined neurologically. New-onset headaches (especially if atypical) and neck stiffness should elicit suspicion. The report recommended that pregnant women with a suspected *stroke* should ideally be admitted to a hyperacute stroke unit.

3.4 MBRRACE-UK report 2015 – highlights and take-home messages

Overview

1. Title of report: ***Saving Lives, Improving Mothers' Care - Surveillance of maternal deaths in the UK 2011–13 and lessons learned to inform maternity care from the UK and Ireland Confidential Enquiries into Maternal Deaths and Morbidity 2009–13.***
2. Topic-specific reviews included: mental health-related causes, VTE, homicide and domestic abuse, cancer and late deaths (between 42 days and 1 year after the end of pregnancy).

Key facts and figures

- The MM rate fell from ten to nine per 100 000 maternities, a statistically significant fall of 35% from 2003–05.
- The leading causes of death were cardiac (*indirect*: $n = 49$; rate 2.09 per 100 000) and VTE (*direct*: $n = 24$; rate 1.01 per 100 000).
- Almost a quarter of *late* maternal deaths (42 days to 1 year after birth) were due to psychiatric causes.
- *Indirect* (medical and psychiatric) deaths remained high. There were no deaths from influenza in 2012–13 (related to a fall in influenza activity, not an increase in vaccination).

Key messages – general

- Of the women who died, the number who delivered in an emergency department or in an ambulance rose from 13% to 18% (3% delivered at home).
- In general, pre-hospital care was of a high standard. There were individual cases where care could have been improved. Examples include:
  - Adrenaline was not given when a breast-feeding woman collapsed despite being indicated.
  - Some interventions were unsuccessful or made the situation worse (e.g. oesophageal intubation).
  - Delay in transporting women to hospital after collapse, with prolonged efforts to resuscitate at the scene (home or other).
  - Poor communication during transport with failure to alert the receiving unit and the receiving obstetrician.
- Access to antenatal care is lacking in women who died, with only one-third receiving the nationally recommended level of care. Many women had recurrent presentations to services, often with escalating symptoms. Recommendation – pre-hospital practitioners should be aware of the increased risk of poor outcome associated with lack of regular antenatal care.

TOP TIP

A timely decision to initiate rapid transfer is required when acute resuscitation is implemented in the pre-hospital situation. During transport ensure clear communication to the receiving unit so that appropriate personnel are on hand on arrival.

Topic-specific key messages – relevant to pre-hospital care

- *Mental health-related causes* – in women who died of mental health causes there was often evidence of poor communication between professional groups and the individuals involved. One in seven women died *by suicide*. Women who died often reported de novo thoughts of violent self-harm, had sudden-onset/rapidly worsening mental symptoms or persistently felt detached from their baby.

> **TOP TIP**
>
> **Seek urgent help from the specialist perinatal mental health team if women describe thoughts of violent self-harm, sudden-onset or rapidly worsening mental symptoms or persistent feelings of detachment from their baby.**

- *Thromboembolism* – more than 80% of women who died from VTE had at least one defined risk factor and 70% had two or more. Also, symptoms and signs were misinterpreted in emergency departments. Recommendation – pre-hospital care practitioners should consider the possibility of VTE in any woman with suggestive symptoms. Assessment should include consideration of all risk factors for VTE.
- *Homicide and domestic abuse* – domestic abuse is more common in pregnancy and the puerperium. A history of previous abuse should alert healthcare professionals to look for symptoms or signs of domestic abuse; the woman will require an opportunity to disclose in a safe environment. Recurrent presentations with unusual symptoms or signs should raise suspicion of domestic abuse.
- *Late deaths* – between 2009 and 2013, 553 women died 42 days to 1 year following pregnancy. Cancer (28%) was the single largest cause. Almost a quarter of late deaths (23%) were associated with long-standing, multiple morbidities persisting after pregnancy, in women leading socially complex lives (14 per 100 000 maternities).

> **TOP TIP**
>
> **Late deaths (>42 days) following pregnancy are associated with long-standing, multiple medical or psychiatric morbidities, in the setting of a complex social background.**

3.5 MBRRACE-UK report 2016 – highlights and take-home messages

Overview

1. Title of report: ***Saving Lives, Improving Mothers' Care – Surveillance of maternal deaths in the UK 2012–14 and lessons learned to inform maternity care from the UK and Ireland Confidential Enquiries into Maternal Deaths and Morbidity 2009–14.***
2. Topic-specific reviews included: cardiovascular disease (including a specific section on women with artificial mechanical heart valves), hypertensive disorders of pregnancy, early pregnancy and critical care.

Key facts and figures

- The MM rate again fell, from 9 to 8.5 per 100 000 maternities.
- *Indirect* (medical and psychiatric) deaths remain high ($n = 119$; rate 5.08 per 100 000) and continued to account for more than two-thirds of all deaths with no significant change from the 2003–05 report.
- The *direct* maternal death rate decreased by 49% between 2003–05 and 2012–14 (RR 0.51, 95% CI 0.38–0.68), a significant trend over time ($p = 0.003$). Although there was a 30% decrease in *indirect* maternal death rate (RR 0.71, 95% CI 0.55–0.90), the trend over time was not statistically significant ($p = 0.093$).
- Cardiac disease remains the commonest cause of *indirect* death and the commonest cause of maternal death overall. Over one-quarter of deaths during pregnancy or up to 42 days afterwards were due to a *cardiovascular* cause ($n = 52$; rate 2.18 per 100 000). Between 2009 and 2014, 189 women died from cardiac causes (108 in pregnancy or within 6 weeks, with an additional 81 *late* deaths).
- Reported successes included:
  - Maternal death rate from hypertensive disease was the lowest ever reported, with *less than one woman in a million* dying from pregnancy-related blood pressure disorder. However, the need or appropriate action when blood pressure is raised is emphasised in the following topic specific section.

- Deaths from influenza reduced dramatically, related primarily to a low level of influenza activity in 2012–14. Increasing immunisation rates in pregnancy remains a public health priority.

Key messages – general

- The WHO re-classified *suicide* as a *direct* cause of maternal death. This is now the leading cause of direct maternal death *occurring within a year after pregnancy*. The MM rate from suicide has not changed since 2003.
- Of the women who died, the number delivered in an emergency department or in an ambulance remained stable at 16% ($n = 22$) (4% ($n = 6$) delivered at home).
- The new *'Three Ps in a Pod'* initiative highlights key messages for emergency services in order to prevent cardiovascular and other indirect maternal deaths. The three 'Ps' represent *'Pregnancy'* ('Think Chest' – cardiac, respiratory, VTE), *'Postnatal'* ('Think Head' – neurological, mental health) and *'Pick up the problem'* ('Think High Risk' – pick up the phone, pick up the problem). A poster is downloadable at https://rcpsg.ac.uk/college/influencing-healthcare/policy/maternal-health (accessed February 2018), and a 5-minute video highlighting the key messages in relation to *indirect* causes of maternal death is also available via the same link.
- Again, many women who died *presented recurrently* to various services, often with escalating symptoms. The report recommends that this should be a 'red flag' triggering appropriate referral and investigation, leading to a definitive diagnosis.

TOP TIP

Escalation or deterioration of symptoms in women who recurrently present to healthcare professionals should be a 'red flag' and referral on for appropriate investigation is recommended.

Topic-specific key messages – relevant to pre-hospital care

- *Cardiovascular disease* – between 2009 and 2014, 153 women died of cardiac-related causes:
  - 77% of those who died had no pre-existing cardiovascular history.
  - Patients who died from cardiac causes often had other medical conditions.
  - The risk of cardiac death is doubled in women aged 35–39 years and is almost four times higher in women >40 years.
  - Sudden arrhythmic cardiac death with a normal heart (sudden adult death syndrome (SADS) ($n = 53$, 35% of cardiac deaths) and ischaemia ($n = 34$, 22% of cardiac deaths) were the commonest causes).
  - Vessel dissection accounted for 32 (20.9%) of cardiac deaths (aortic dissection ($n = 21$, 13.7%) and coronary dissection ($n = 11$, 7.2%)).
  - Almost one in five of these women died in an ambulance or emergency department.
- The report recommends that ambulance and emergency department staff must be aware of the following:
  - The possibility of undiagnosed cardiac disease in pregnant or recently delivered women.
  - That *persistent* breathlessness or orthopnoea (breathlessness on lying flat) is abnormal in pregnancy and may indicate a significant cardiovascular problem.
- That *severe* chest pain spreading to the left arm or back may be cardiac in origin.
- That a normal ECG (and/or a negative troponin) does not exclude the diagnosis of an acute coronary syndrome.
- The appropriate modifications to resuscitation needed in pregnancy, including manual uterine displacement or left lateral tilt, early intubation with a cuffed tracheal tube and early recourse to PMCS. There were several cases where extensive and prolonged resuscitation attempts were made prior to transfer to hospital. PMCS is a vital part of maternal resuscitation and prompt transfer is needed to enable this to take place.

TOP TIP

Cardiac disease is the commonest cause of maternal death and symptoms suggestive of cardiac disease should not be ignored.

TOP TIP

A normal ECG (and/or a negative troponin) does not exclude acute coronary syndrome.

- *Women with artificial heart valves* are at extremely high risk of developing complications in pregnancy. Symptoms may develop for the first time during pregnancy because of the physiological increase in cardiac output. This is a particular risk for those with *valvular stenosis*. Full anticoagulation with low molecular weight heparin (LMWH) is required for those with prosthetic valves.
- *Hypertensive disorders of pregnancy* – several recommendations were made relevant to pre-hospital care:
  - Blood pressure should be recorded regularly in both primary and secondary care. These results should be available to pre-hospital care practitioners within patient-held maternity records.
  - Blood pressure should be kept below 150/100 mmHg to reduce the risk of intracerebral bleeding.

TOP TIP

If blood pressure in labour or immediately after birth is above 140 mmHg systolic or 90 mmHg diastolic on two occasions, transfer to a consultant obstetric unit should be arranged.

- *Early pregnancy* – there were 12 deaths from early pregnancy causes in 2009–14, and nine (75%) were due to ruptured ectopic pregnancy. Three deaths (25%) were related to termination of pregnancy (including one illegal self-induced termination). The incidence of ectopic pregnancy is 11 per 1000 pregnancies, with almost 12 000 women per year diagnosed in the UK. Eight of the nine women who died as a result of ectopic pregnancy presented with haemodynamic collapse. Recommendation – *ruptured ectopic pregnancy* should always be considered in any woman of reproductive age presenting with collapse, dizziness, acute abdominal/pelvic pain or gastrointestinal symptoms (including diarrhoea or vomiting), regardless of whether pregnancy has been confirmed.

TOP TIP

If a woman of reproductive age presents with shock or collapse in the community, with no obvious cause, institute immediate resuscitation and transfer without delay to a hospital emergency department for urgent assessment and treatment.

- *Critical care* – several recommendations made in this section are pertinent to care in the pre-hospital care setting:
  - Early recognition of critical illness is vitally important – raised respiratory rate, persistent tachycardia, chest pain and orthopnoea are important signs and symptoms which should always be fully investigated. Rapid transfer to an emergency department is recommended.
  - Reduced or altered conscious level is not an early warning sign; it is a 'red flag', often indicating an established illness.

3.6 MBRRACE-UK report 2017 – highlights and take-home messages

Overview

1. Title of report: ***Saving Lives, Improving Mothers' Care – Lessons learned to inform maternity care from the UK and Ireland Confidential Enquiries into Maternal Deaths and Morbidity 2013–15***.
2. Topic-specific reviews included: deaths from epilepsy, deaths from haemorrhage, amniotic fluid embolism (AFE), anaesthesia, stroke, respiratory, endocrine and other indirect causes, severe morbidity from psychosis.

Key facts and figures

- The MM rate rose for the first time to 8.8 per 100 000 maternities, although this was only a slight increase and still ostensibly a decreasing overall trend.
- Two-thirds of women who died had pre-existing physical or mental health problems.
- *Indirect* deaths remain high (*n* = 114; rate 4.94 per 100 000) and continued to account for more than two-thirds of all deaths with no significant change from the 2003–05 report.

- Cardiac disease remained the leading cause of indirect maternal death during or up to 6 weeks after the end of pregnancy with a rate of 2.34 per 100 000 maternities
- The rates of overall mortality and direct maternal death in the 2013–15 triennium were not significantly different from the rates in 2010–12. However, the indirect maternal death rate was significantly lower in 2013–15 than 2010–12
- Maternal suicide is the third largest cause of direct maternal deaths occurring during or within 42 days of the end of pregnancy. However, it remains the leading cause of direct deaths occurring during pregnancy or up to a year after the end of pregnancy, with one in seven women who die in the period between 6 weeks and 1 year after pregnancy dying by suicide.
- One of the most marked observations is the dramatic decrease in the rates of maternal death from sepsis due to indirect causes, not only due to a decrease in influenza-related maternal deaths, but also due to a decrease in maternal deaths from causes such as pneumonia and meningitis.

Key messages – general

- High-level actions are needed to ensure that it is seen as the responsibility of all health professionals to facilitate opportunistic pre- and post-pregnancy counselling and appropriate framing of the advice when women with pre-existing conditions attend any appointment, and that resources for pre- and post-pregnancy counselling are provided, together with open access to specialist contraceptive services.
- Women with epilepsy should be provided, before conception, with verbal and written information on prenatal screening and its implications, the risks of self-discontinuation of antiepileptic drugs and the effects of seizures and antiepileptics on the fetus and on the pregnancy, breastfeeding and contraception.
- Women with any past history of psychotic disorder, even where not diagnosed as postpartum psychosis or bipolar disorder, should be regarded as at elevated risk in future postpartum periods and should be referred to mental health services in pregnancy to receive an individualised assessment of risk.
- Women should be advised, within 24 hours of giving birth, of the symptoms and signs of conditions, including sepsis, that may threaten their lives and require them to access emergency treatment.

Topic-specific key messages – relevant to pre-hospital care

- When assessing a woman who is unwell, consider her clinical condition in addition to her MEOWS score.
- Midwives and others carrying out postnatal checks in the community should have a thermometer to enable them to check the temperature of women who are unwell.
- Pregnancy should not alter the investigation and treatment of a woman presenting with a stroke.
- Consideration should be given to 'declaring sepsis', analogous to activation of the major obstetric haemorrhage protocol, to ensure the relevant members of the multidisciplinary team are informed, aware and act.
- Neurological examination including assessment for neck stiffness and fundoscopy is mandatory for all women with new-onset headaches or headaches with atypical features, particularly focal symptoms.
- In sudden-onset severe maternal shock, e.g. anaphylaxis, the presence of a pulse may be an unreliable indicator of adequate cardiac output. In the absence of a recordable blood pressure or other indicator of cardiac output, the early initiation of external cardiac compressions may be life-saving.
- In cases of massive obstetric haemorrhage, women must be adequately resuscitated and bleeding stopped prior to extubation following general anaesthesia. Evidence of adequate resuscitation should be sought prior to extubation.
- Aortocaval compression should be suspected in any supine pregnant woman who develops severe hypotension after induction of anaesthesia, even if some lateral tilt has been applied. If there is a delay in delivery, putting the woman into the left lateral position may be the only option if other manoeuvres fail or if the woman has refractory severe hypotension.
- The choice of endotracheal tube for pregnant women should start at size 7.0 mm and proceed to smaller tube selections if needed (size 6.0 and 5.0 mm). It is recommended that all resuscitation carts used in maternity units should include endotracheal tubes no larger than 7.0 mm and include smaller sizes such as 6.0 and 5.0 mm.
- Haemorrhage should be considered when classic signs of hypovolaemia are present (tachycardia and/or agitation and the late sign of hypotension) even in the absence of revealed bleeding.

Summary of key points

- The Confidential Enquiry into Maternal Deaths (CEMD) is now part of the MBRRACE-UK programme that produces detailed annual reports, examining the underlying causes of pregnancy-related deaths throughout the UK and Ireland, with recommendations for improving practice
- Each annual report will continue to include focused, topic-specific reviews
- All pre-hospital care practitioners must:
  - Have a thorough knowledge of normal physiology and common pathologies in pregnancy
  - Be aware that *indirect causes* are the major contributor to maternal death in the UK and Ireland (cardiac, non-genital sepsis, neurological and psychiatric)
  - Ensure rapid assessment and intervention at the scene for pregnancy emergencies, but remain aware when to initiate rapid transfer
  - Carefully consider which facility is most appropriate for transfer to, ensuring appropriate medical staffing and resource will be available (e.g. obstetric, neonatal, accident and emergency, trauma). This will depend on the specific pregnancy complication and the clinical state of the woman and/or her baby
  - Be aware of the importance of clear communication with the woman and her family and all practitioners involved in the care of the pregnancy-related emergency:
    - Midwives in community, maternity unit and hospital settings
    - Emergency department staff and also obstetricians in cases of collapse in pregnancy
    - Ambulance control centres
  - Be aware that late pregnancy-related deaths (>42 days after the birth) are associated with long-term medical and psychiatric morbidities in women with often complex social lives
- All pre-hospital care practitioners should visit the MBRRACE-UK website each December to review the annual updates – https://www.npeu.ox.ac.uk/mbrrace-uk (accessed February 2018)

CHAPTER 4

Getting it right – non-technical skills and communications

Learning outcomes

After reading this chapter, you will be able to:
- Describe how human factors affect the performance of individuals and teams in the healthcare environment

4.1 Introduction

The emphasis on the management of obstetric emergency care has traditionally concentrated on the knowledge of the treatment process, for example, when to give a specific intervention, drug or aliquot of fluid. An often overlooked element is how in these high-pressure situations individuals from a variety of different professional and specialty backgrounds come together to form an effective team that minimises errors and works actively to prevent adverse events

This chapter provides a brief introduction to some of the human factors that can affect the performance of individuals and teams in the healthcare environment. Human factors, also referred to as ergonomics, is an established scientific discipline and clinical human factors has been described as:

> Enhancing clinical performance through an understanding of the effects of teamwork, tasks, equipment, workspace, culture and organisation on human behaviour and abilities and application of that knowledge in clinical settings.
>
> (Catchpole, 2010)

4.2 Extent of healthcare error

In 2000, an influential report entitled *To Err is Human: Building a safer health system* (Kohn et al., 2000) suggested that across the United States somewhere between 44000 and 98000 deaths each year could be attributed to medical error. A pilot study in the UK demonstrated that approximately one in ten patients admitted to healthcare experienced an adverse event.

Healthcare has been able to learn from a number of other high-risk industries, including the nuclear, petrochemical, space exploration, military and aviation industries, about how team issues have been managed. These lessons have been slowly adopted and translated to healthcare.

Specialist working groups and national bodies have been instrumental in promoting awareness of the importance of human factors in healthcare. They aim to raise awareness and promote the principles and practices of human factors, identify current human factor activity, capability and barriers, and create conditions to support human factors being embedded at a local

Pre-Obstetric Emergency Training: A Practical Approach, Second Edition. Edited by Mark Woolcock.
© 2019 John Wiley & Sons Ltd. Published 2019 by John Wiley & Sons Ltd.

level. One such example of this in the UK is the Human Factors Clinical Working Group and the National Quality Board's concordat statement on human factors.

4.3 Causes of healthcare error

Consider this example of an adverse event:

A woman needs to receive an infusion of a particular drug. An error occurs and the woman receives an incorrect drug. What are the potential causes of this situation?

Potential causes of our example drug error	
Prescription error	Wrong drug prescribed
Preparation error	Correct drug prescribed but misread
Preparation error	Contents mislabelled during manufacture
Drawing up error	Incorrect drug selected
Administration error	Patient ID mix-up, drug given to wrong patient

Q. What one thing links all of these errors?
A. The humans involved – these are all examples of human errors.

Humans make mistakes. No amount of checks and procedures will mitigate this fact. In fact the only way to completely remove human error is to remove all the humans involved. It is vital therefore that we look to work in a way that, wherever possible, minimises the occurrence of mistakes and ensures that when they do occur the method minimises the chance of it resulting in an adverse event.

4.4 Human error

It has been suggested that these human errors can be further categorised into: (i) those that occur at the sharp end of care by the treating team and individuals; and (ii) those that occur at a blunt or organisational level, typically through policies, procedures, staffing and culture.

These errors can be further subdivided as shown in Table 4.1.

Table 4.1 Types of errors		Explanation	Example
Sharp errors that occur with the team/individuals treating the patient	Mistake	Lack or misapplication of knowledge	Not knowing the correct drug to prescribe
	Slip or lapse	Skills-based mistake	Knowing the correct drug but writing another one
	Violation	Deliberate action that may be routine or exceptional	Not attempting to get a drug second checked as there are no staff available
Blunt/organisational errors		Policies, procedures, infrastructure and building layout that has errors embedded	Different drugs used by different specialities and departments for same condition

It is typically found that the latent/organisational issues often coexist with the sharp errors; in fact it is rare for an isolated error to occur – often there is a chain of events that results in the adverse event. The 'Swiss cheese' model demonstrates how apparently random, unconnected events and organisational decisions can all make errors more likely (Figure 4.1). Conversely, a standardised system with good defence mechanisms can capture these errors and prevent adverse events.

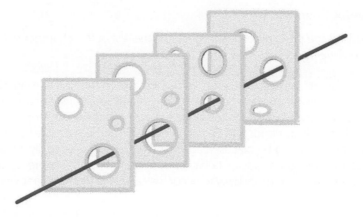

Figure 4.1 The 'Swiss cheese' model

Each of the slices of Swiss cheese represents barriers that, under ideal circumstances, would prevent or detect the error. The holes represent weaknesses in these barriers; if the holes align, the error passes through undetected.

Reconsider the example of drug error using the Swiss cheese model. The first slice is the practitioner writing the prescription, the second slice is the organisation's drug policy, the third is the practitioner who draws up the drug and the fourth is the practitioner who second checks the drug.

Now consider the following: What if the first practitioner is very junior and not familiar with that area or the drugs used? – her slice of cheese has larger holes. What if the organisation has failed to develop a robust drug policy that is fit for purpose? – this second slice is considerably weakened or may even be removed completely. What if the practitioner does not normally work on that ward and is not familiar with the commonly used drugs? – his slice has also got larger holes. What if this area is always short of staff, so staff do not routinely attempt to get the drug second checked? – this slice is completely removed.

The end result is that multiple defences have been weakened or removed and error is more likely, and the error is more likely to cause harm. Also be aware of the different types of error with potential gaps in knowledge, a latent/organisational error (no effective policy and possibly an issue with nurse staffing) and a routine violation.

4.5 Learning from error

Historically, those making mistakes have been identified and singled out for punishment and/or retraining, in what is often referred to as a culture of blame. With our example, drug error blame would most likely have fallen on the shoulders of the nurse administering and/or the doctor incorrectly prescribing. Does retraining these individuals make it safer for other or future patients? That clearly depends on the underlying reasons. If it was purely a knowledge gap, possibly, but does the same knowledge gap exist elsewhere? Potentially all the other issues remain unresolved. Moreover such punitive reactions make it less likely for individuals to admit mistakes and near misses in the future.

The focus is now on learning from error and in shifting away from the individual, is much more focused on determining the system/organisational errors. Once robust systems, procedures and policies that work and are effective are in place, then errors can be captured. Of course, issues will still need to be addressed where individuals have been reckless or lacked knowledge – but now reasons why the individuals felt the need to violate procedures or had not been given all the knowledge required, can be looked at.

For this to work health services need to learn from errors, adverse events and near misses. This requires engagement at both the individual level, by reporting errors, and the organisational level, investigating and feeding back the error using a systematic approach. It is also key that information is cascaded through the organisation and across the health service to raise awareness and prevent similar situations occurring.

Violation may be indicative of the failure of systems, procedures or policies or other cultural issues. It is important that policies, procedures, roles and even our buildings and equipment are all designed proactively with human factors in mind so things do not have to be fixed retrospectively when adverse events occur. This means that all members of the organisation must be aware of human factors, not just the front-line clinical staff.

Improving team and individual performance

Having discussed the magnitude of the problem of healthcare error, the rest of this chapter will focus on how the team and individuals' performance can be developed.

Raising awareness of the human factors in healthcare error, and being able to practise relevant skills and behaviours within multi-professional teams allows the development of effective teams in all situations. Simulation activity allows a team to explore these new ideas, practise them and develop them. To do this we need feedback on our performance within a safe environment where no patient is at risk and egos and personal interests can be set aside. Consider how you developed a clinical skill. It was something that needed to be practised again and again until eventually it started to become automatic and routine. The same applies for our human factor behaviours. In addition, through recognising our inherent human limitations and the situations when errors are more likely to occur we can all be hypervigilant when required.

4.6 Communication

Poor communication is the leading cause of adverse events. This is not surprising; to have an effective team there needs to be good communication. The leader needs to communicate with the followers, and followers communicate with the leaders and other followers. Communication is not just saying something – it is ensuring that information is accurately passed on and received. We all want to ensure effective communication at all times. Remember there are multiple components to effective communication (Table 4.2).

Table 4.2 Elements of communication				
Sender	**Sender**	**Transmitted**	**Receiver**	**Receiver**
Thinks of what to say	Says message	Through air, over phone, via email	Hears it	Thinks about it and acts

When communicating face-to-face a lot of the information is transmitted non-verbally, which can make telephone or email conversations more challenging. Communication can be more difficult when talking across professional, specialty or hierarchal barriers as we do not always talk the same technical language, have the same levels of understanding, or even have a full awareness of the other person's role.

There are a variety of similar tools to aid communication, such as SBAR (situation, background, assessment and recommendation). Find out what tool your organisation has in place and practise using it; look out for other staff using it too. SBAR is designed for acute clinical communications. It facilitates the sender to plan and organise the message, make it succinct and focused, and provide it in a logical and expected order. It is also an empowerment tool allowing the sender (who may be more junior) to request an action from a more senior individual. While these tools are useful, they tend to be reserved for certain situations, whilst we want to establish effective communication as the routine not the exception. One method to routinely improve communication is to incorporate a feedback loop.

Effective communication with a feedback loop

Errors can occur at any level or at multiple levels. Consider a busy clinical situation and the team leader shouts '*We need an ECG connecting*' while looking at the blood pressure – what happens? The majority of times nothing – nobody goes to connect the ECG! So how can this be improved? Most obviously, an individual can be identified to perform the task, by name: '*Mark can you please connect the ECG?*' If Mark says '*yes*' effective communication might be assumed, but this is not always the case. What has Mark heard and what will he do? At the moment we do not really know what message has been received. Mark might dash over with a cup of tea, as this is what he thought he heard. This may seem a slightly strange thing to happen, but how often in a clinical emergency have you asked for something and been presented with something else? People are less likely to ask questions in emergencies as everyone is busy. This could be the catalyst for an error or could precipitate a missed task. So how do we find out what message Mark received? The easiest way is to include a feedback loop.

> Now the conversation goes:
>
> Team leader: '*Mark, can you please connect the ECG?*'
> Mark: '*Okay, just connecting the ECG*'

We now know that the message has been transmitted and received correctly. For this process to work both parties (the sender and receiver) need to understand and expect it – again demonstrating the need for us to practise and train together.

4.7 Team working, leadership and followership

At a basic level a team is a group of individuals with a common cause. Historically, we have tended to train individually or in professional silos; the risk here is that we are making a 'team of experts' rather than an 'expert team'. Often, within healthcare, our teams form at short notice and often arrive at different times. Much emphasis has previously been given to the role of the leader, but a leader cannot be a team on his or her own. As much emphasis should be given to developing the other team members, the active followers. A good leader will be able to swap from the role of leader to follower as more senior staff arrive and agree to take over.

The leader

The leader's role is multifaceted and includes directing the team, assigning tasks and assessing performance, motivating and encouraging the team to work together, and planning and organising. All leadership skills and behaviours need to be developed and practised. There are different leadership styles and the leader needs to choose an appropriate style for that situation. Effective communication is key, and should be reviewed and reflected upon regularly. Constructive feedback should both be given and sought in order to facilitate continuously improving performance.

Who is the leader?

It is vitally important to have a clearly identified leader. There can be times when people come and go, or different specialties arrive, creating a situation where it may not be clear who the leader is. In some situations or institutions, individuals will wear tabards or other forms of identification to mitigate against this uncertainty. If there is a scribe recording events, they should record who is leading and any changes to the leadership.

Physical position of the leader

As soon as the leader becomes hands-on and task focused, they are primarily concentrating on the task at hand. This becomes the focus of their thoughts and they lose situation awareness and their objective overview of the situation. The leader should be standing in an optimal position where they can gather all the information and ideally view the patient, the team members and the monitoring and diagnostic equipment. This enables them to recognise when a member is struggling with a task or procedure and support them appropriately.

Clear roles

Ideally, the team should meet before the event and have the opportunity to introduce each other, and clarify roles and actions in emergencies. Sometimes this can be facilitated at the beginning of a shift, but at other times it is impossible to predict or arrange. It is important, therefore, that individuals identify themselves to the leader as they arrive and roles are agreed, allocated and understood. A lot of the time their role may be determined purely in relation to the specific bleep the individual carries, but it is important that team members are flexible, e.g. if three airway providers were first on scene we would expect other tasks to also be undertaken.

Followership

The followers have roles that are as mission critical as the leader's role. Followers are expected to work within their scope of practice and take the initiative. No one would expect to turn up at a ward emergency and have a neat row of staff against the wall waiting for instructions. It is important to think about the level of communication required between the leader and followers. If it is obvious a task is being done, this does not need to communicated. There is a risk that followers can overwhelm the leader with verbal communications when, in fact, the key is to communicate concerns or abnormal things. In the Formula One pit lane during a tyre change, the crew communicate (visually) as tasks are completed; they also signal if they have a problem, but they do not communicate every expected step.

Hierarchy

Within the team there needs to be a hierarchy. This is the power gradient; the leader is at the top of this, as the person coordinating, directing and making the decisions. However, this should not be absolute. There is much discussion in the literature about the degree of the hierarchical gradient. If it is too steep, the leader has a massive position of power, his decisions are unquestionable and the followers blindly follow his orders. This is not safe because leaders are humans too and also make errors – their team is their safety net. Safe practice is achieved where the followers feel they can raise concerns or question instructions. This must always be understood by the leaders as much as by the followers. One way to reduce the hierarchy is for the leader to invite the team's thoughts and concerns, particularly around patient safety issues. It is also important for the follower to learn how to raise concerns appropriately.

One method that is sometimes used to raise concerns appropriately is PACE (probing, alerting, challenging or declaring an emergency). The probing question allows diplomacy and maintenance of the hierarchy whilst raising a point.

Stage	Level of concern
P – Probe	*I think you need to know what is happening*
A – Alert	*I think something bad might happen*
C – Challenge	*I know something bad will happen*
E – Emergency	*I will not let it happen*

These stages are described with examples:

- **Probe** – this is used where a person notices something they think might be a problem. They verbalise the issue, often as a question. 'Have you noticed that this child is cyanosed?'
- **Alert** – the observer strengthens and directs their statement and suggests a course of action. 'Dr Davis, I am concerned, the child is deeply cyanosed, should we start BVM ventilation?'
- **Challenge** – the situation requires urgent attention. One of the key protagonists needs to be directly engaged. If possible the speaker places his- or herself into the eye line of the person they wish to communicate with. 'Dr Davis, you must listen to me now, this patient needs help with his ventilation.'
- **Emergency** – this is used where all else has failed and/or the observer perceives a critical event is about to occur. Where possible a physical signal or physical barrier should be employed together with clear verbalisation. 'Dr Davis, you are overlooking this child's respiratory state, please move out of the way I am going to ventilate him.'

The PACE structure can be commenced at any appropriate level and escalated until a satisfactory response is gained. If an adverse event is imminent then it may be relevant to start at the declaring 'emergency' stage, whereas a much lower level of concern may well start at a 'probing' question.

Some industries have additionally adopted organisation-wide critical phrases that convey the importance of the situation, e.g. 'I am concerned', 'I am uncomfortable' or 'I am scared'.

4.8 Situation awareness

A key element of good team working and leadership is to be fully aware of what is happening; this is termed situation awareness. It not only involves seeing what is happening but also captures how this is interpreted and understood, how decisions are made and ultimately to plan ahead.

Typically, three levels of situation awareness are described:

Level 1 – What is going on?
Level 2 – So what?
Level 3 – Now what?

Consider **level 1** – the basic level – we are prone to errors even at this level. This is an active process; the risk seen is what one expects to see, rather than what is actually there. Figure 4.2 shows the similar package design of two different medications, making errors more likely. It is important to really concentrate on seeing what is there in reality.

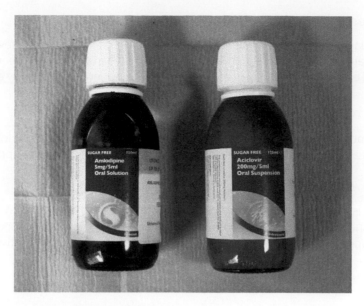

Figure 4.2 Similar package design of two different medications

Distraction

Within healthcare, distractions become the norm to such an extent individuals are often not even aware of them. The risk is that mistakes are made and information is missed. It is important to try to challenge interruptions when doing critical tasks, and when they do occur restart the task from the beginning, rather than from where it is considered the interruption occurred. Some organisations have set aside specific quiet areas for critical tasks. Whatever the local set up, the key is to develop and maintain everyone's awareness of how distraction greatly increases the chance of error.

Level 2 captures how someone's understanding forms from what has been seen. To minimise level 2 errors consideration is needed as to how the human brain works, recognises things and makes decisions and choices. This level of detail is beyond the scope of this introductory chapter, and therefore this section will focus on a part of this – the decision making that leads into level 3.

On the face of it the practice of decision making is familiar to everyone. However, to understand the factors that can compromise this process, it is important to understand the factors that will influence the decision made. To make a good decision a person needs to assess all aspects of a problem, identify the possible responses to the problem, consider the consequences of each of those responses and then weigh up the advantages and disadvantages in order to draw a conclusion. Having completed this, they then need to communicate their decision to their team.

Good situation awareness is a basic prerequisite of this process. To achieve this, the decision maker must ensure they have all the key information. The whole team should be on the alert for ambiguities or conflicting information. Any inconsistent facts should be treated as a potential marker for faulty situation awareness; they should never be brushed off as unimportant anomalies in the absence of evidence to support such a decision.

In many clinical situations there can be a significant pressure of time. Where this is not the case then no decision-making process should be concluded until the team is satisfied they have all the information and have considered all the options. Where time is under pressure, a certain amount of pragmatism must be employed. There is plenty of evidence to confirm that practise and experience can mitigate some of the negative effects of abbreviating a decision-making process. Those making decisions under such circumstances need to remain aware of the short-cuts they have taken. They should be ready to receive feedback from their team, particularly if any member of the team has significant concerns about the proposed course of action.

Level 3 – having seen and understood we can now plan forward and communicate this with the team.

Team situation awareness

The individuals in the team may have a differing awareness of the situation depending on their previous experiences, specialty, physical position, etc. The team's situation awareness will often be greater than that of any one individual, but this can only be exploited if the individual elements are effectively communicated. The leader should actively encourage this.

4.9 Improving team and individual performance

In addition to effective communication, team working, situation awareness and leadership and followership skills, there are a number of other ways that team and individual performance can be further developed and improved.

Awareness of situations when errors are more likely

If we are aware that an error is more likely we can be more proactive in detecting them. Two common situations that make errors more likely are stress and fatigue. Stress is not only a source of error when we are overworked and overstimulated, but also at the other end of the spectrum – when we are understimulated we can become inattentive.

The acronym HALT has been used to describe situations when error is more likely:

H – Hungry
A – Angry
L – Late
T – Tired

IMSAFE has been used as a checklist in the aviation industry, asking whether the individual may be affected by:

I – Illness
M – Medication
S – Stress
A – Alcohol
F – Fatigue
E – Eating

Ideally, individuals who are potentially compromised need to be supported appropriately, allowed time to recover and the team made aware of the situation. How this can be achieved in the middle of a night shift can be problematic.

Awareness of error traps

A common trap that people fall into is only seeing or registering the information that fits in with their current mental model. This is known as a *confirmation bias*. When this occurs people favour information that confirms their preconceptions or hypotheses regardless of whether the information is true. This may be observed within the healthcare setting during the process of a referral or handover. An example of this might be a clinician receiving a phone call requesting them to attend the ward to review an acutely deteriorating patient. The clinician is advised that the patient is known to have asthma. On their way to the ward the clinician builds up a series of preconceived expectations around what they will find upon their arrival. They may even formulate a management plan whilst travelling to the scene, based upon their expectations. Once this mindset is established it can be difficult to shift.

On arrival, the clinician examines the systems affected by the presumed diagnosis. They seek to confirm their expectation by focusing on an auscultation of the chest at the expense of a thorough assessment. Upon hearing bilateral wheeze their preconceived ideas are confirmed and the remainder of the assessment is completed without due attention and more as a rehearsed exercise than an open-minded exploration. They fail to notice that the patient also has a soft stridor and is hypotensive. In this case the eventual diagnosis of anaphylaxis becomes at best a very late consideration, or at worst a situation that requires an objective newcomer to the team to point out the obvious.

Cognitive aids: checklists, guidelines and protocols

Cognitive aids such as guidelines are important because the human memory is not infallible. They also improve team understanding through the use of a standardised response. This reduces stress. This is especially true where an uncommon emergency event occurs. The team may be unfamiliar with one another and each member will be trying to remember what to do, what treatments are required and in what order. A good team leader will use the available cognitive aids as a prompt and the team's members can use it as a resource so that they can plan ahead. Safe practice is promoted through the use of these tools in an emergency rather than relying on memory.

Calling for help early

Trainee staff are often reluctant to call for senior help, partly due to not recognising the severity of the situation but also due to concerns about wasting the time of seniors. With all emergency events, and in particular with paediatric emergencies, escalation and appropriate help should be summoned as soon as possible. Remember help will not arrive instantly.

Using all available resources

Team resources include staff, observations, equipment, cognitive aids and the facilities in the local area. The team leader should continually consider the appropriateness of utilising available un-tasked staff or equipment to optimise the patient's care and prevent a bottleneck in the treatment pathway.

Debriefing

Wherever possible a debriefing should be facilitated, even if briefly, following clinical events. Ideally this should be normal procedure rather than being reserved for catastrophic events. The aim of a debrief is to summarise any particular issues or problems that the team had, and reflect on how the team performed. Some organisations have set templates to facilitate this. It gives the opportunity for individuals, teams and organisations to continually develop.

Summary of key points

- Human factors can lead to poor team working, patient harm and adverse events
- It is really important for you to use every opportunity to reflect and develop your own performance and influence the development of others and the team
- Appropriate debriefing is included in the scenarios for the POET course; these may be incorporated into your own clinical practice

CHAPTER 5
Anatomical and physiological changes in pregnancy

Learning outcomes

After reading this chapter, you will be able to:
- Describe the anatomical and physiological changes in the airway, breathing, circulatory, genital tract and gastrointestinal systems during pregnancy and their implications for management
- State the correct positioning of a patient >20 weeks' pregnant
- Recognise common laboratory test results in pregnancy

5.1 Anatomical and physiological changes in pregnancy and implications for management

Airway

Although the airway itself does not change dramatically as a result of pregnancy, other anatomical and physiological changes will result in the need to modify priorities and strategies for airway management. Increasing numbers of obstetric patients are morbidly obese, and this creates further management issues with the airway (Heslehurst et al., 2007). In the triennium 2013–15, 34% of all the women who died from direct or indirect causes were obese (MBRRACE-UK, 2017).

The neck may appear short and obese, and the obstetric patient is likely to have engorged breasts, particularly in late pregnancy. If the patient is suffering from a hypertensive disorder, oedema of the upper airway may be present. Obstetric patients tend to be young and therefore are likely to have full dentition.

Physiological changes in the gastrointestinal system can also have significant implications for airway management. In the patient with a reduced conscious level, the risk of regurgitation, aspiration and Mendelson's syndrome (an acute chemical pneumonitis caused by the aspiration of stomach contents) increases due to a combination of factors:

- A relaxed gastro-oesophageal sphincter
- Increased intragastric pressure
- Delayed gastric emptying due to upward pressure on the diaphragm from the gravid uterus (again, particularly in the third trimester)

Pre-Obstetric Emergency Training: A Practical Approach, Second Edition. Edited by Mark Woolcock.
© 2019 John Wiley & Sons Ltd. Published 2019 by John Wiley & Sons Ltd.

> **TOP TIP**
>
> Early airway management (either with a supraglottic airway (SGA) or intubation) is essential in the pregnant patient without a gag reflex.

Breathing

In late pregnancy the tidal volume increases by 20% at 12 weeks and by 30–50% at 40 weeks. Because the total lung capacity is unchanged, this increase in tidal volume is at the expense of a proportionate decrease in inspiratory and expiratory reserve, and residual capacity is decreased by up to 25%. Therefore, the patient will have a reduced ability to compensate for any increase in oxygen demand due to illness or injury.

Indeed, the normal physiological demands of pregnancy result in an increase in oxygen demand of 20% in the well obstetric patient. This is met by a small increase in respiratory rate of approximately 1–2 breaths per minute as well as the increased tidal volume.

The shape of the rib cage changes, splaying out at its base due to the need to accommodate a gravid uterus. This reduces costal excursion and so the diaphragm plays an increasingly significant role in supporting respiration as the pregnancy progresses.

During labour and delivery there is an increase in hyperventilation due to pain and anxiety, and in particular during the effort exerted during the second stage of labour.

> **TOP TIP**
>
> Pregnant women have little respiratory reserve. Monitor oxygen saturation and give oxygen immediately if saturation on air falls below 94%. If SpO_2 is less than 85% use a non-rebreathing mask; otherwise use a simple face mask. Aim for a target saturation of 94–98%.

Circulation

Blood volume rises throughout pregnancy, and by the last trimester it will have increased by up to 50%. This increase can be even greater in women with a multiple pregnancy. Red blood cell numbers also rise, but since this is to a lesser degree than plasma volumes, the actual haemoglobin concentration falls. This results in a dilutional anaemia (or haemodilution) compared with the non-pregnant state, and a subsequent reduced capacity for carrying oxygen.

By the middle of pregnancy, cardiac output rises by approximately 40% due largely to an increase in the stroke volume. This is also due, to a lesser extent, to an increase in the pulse rate to about 85–100 bpm at the end of the third trimester. However, the workload of the heart is not increased due to the reduction in blood viscosity (as a result of haemodilution) and decreased peripheral vascular resistance (reduced afterload).

> **TOP TIP**
>
> Extrasystoles are common in pregnancy and are usually harmless.

Cardiac output increases due to:

- Hormone-mediated peripheral vasodilatation
- Greater metabolic requirements arising from increased organ size and activity (particularly relating to the lungs, kidneys, gastrointestinal system and skin)
- Increased heat production (resulting in vasodilatation in the skin)
- The placenta's function as a shunt between the arterial and venous systems (the lack of a capillary system where branches of the uterine artery connect directly to the placental venous sinuses results in a lowered peripheral resistance)

The reduction in peripheral vascular resistance places obstetric patients at risk of postural hypotension due to the potential for a sudden drop in systolic blood pressure when moving to a standing position. This may result in cerebral hypoperfusion and, consequently, syncope. To avoid this risk, obstetric patients should be encouraged to move from a lying to sitting or sitting to standing position slowly. For example, if they are moving from lying to standing they should:

- Sit up with their legs out straight
- Wait for a few seconds and then check for dizziness
- Move so that their legs are bent over the edge of the bed
- Wait for a few seconds and then check for dizziness
- Stand up

At the beginning of pregnancy, the systolic blood pressure falls, but returns to near normal levels at term. Despite this, the pulse pressure increases due to a relatively greater fall in diastolic pressure. As in all patients, the systolic blood pressure provides a more useful indicator of patient status than the diastolic, with the exception that diastolic pressure is as important as systolic pressure in hypertension. The diastolic pressure should be documented at the point the sounds disappear (Korotkoff phase V). Occasionally in pregnancy, the sounds may not disappear. In that circumstance, diastolic blood pressure can be estimated by noting when the sounds become muffled (Korotkoff phase IV) (see Chapter 6).

Varicose veins often occur in the legs due to an increase in venous pressure, relaxation of the smooth muscle of the veins due to the effects of progesterone, and the presence of peripheral oedema. Changes in blood viscosity, venous stasis and impaired venous return during pregnancy increase the risk of venous thromboembolism.

During the late second and third trimester of pregnancy, if the patient lays flat on her back, the gravid uterus can result in supine hypotension due to aortocaval compression. The weight of the uterus compresses the inferior vena cava reducing venous return, in turn reducing cardiac filling and causing a fall in cardiac output. In response, arterial vasoconstriction occurs but arterial pressure will nevertheless fall if vena caval compression is not rapidly corrected, and the resulting low intra-aortic pressure will allow the aorta to be compressed. The effect on the patient is maternal syncope due to reduced cerebral perfusion, and fetal hypoxia due to uterine hypoperfusion. In pre-existing low-output states such as hypovolaemic shock or chest compressions during cardiac arrest, the net result may be little or no maternal and fetal circulation.

After 20 weeks of pregnancy women should NEVER be laid flat on their back. Encourage a position of comfort (semi-recumbent) or full left lateral position for conscious patients (Figure 5.1).

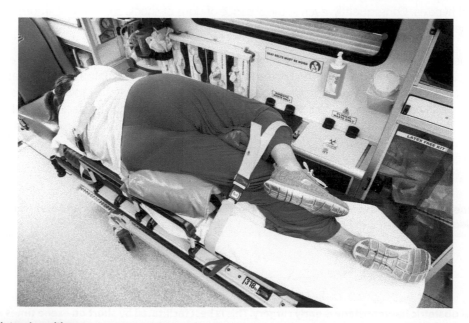

Figure 5.1 Full left lateral position

TOP TIP

In some ambulances, a patient placed on her left will face the saloon wall, thus in these situations, a right lateral position is reasonable (Figure 5.2).

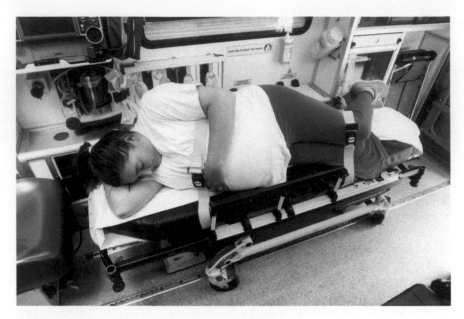

Figure 5.2 Patient in RIGHT lateral position to avoid facing saloon wall

In the event of hypovolaemic shock, the normal physiological changes of pregnancy (increased plasma and red cell volume) allow the patient to compensate for some time. This can make diagnosis difficult, as changes in vital signs may be minimal. Instead, the practitioner must rely on identifying external blood loss or by having a high index of suspicion for internal concealed haemorrhage.

The main mechanism of maintaining maternal circulation in the event of blood loss is the restriction of blood flow to the uterus. This can occur rapidly following the onset of significant bleeding, and will result in a reduction in placental perfusion with associated fetal hypoxia. Consequently, even in the absence of signs of shock, control of haemorrhage and restoration of circulating volume have the highest priority.

If blood loss continues there are few other compensatory mechanisms remaining, since stroke volume is already increased as a normal physiological change of pregnancy. Although the heart rate may rise, this has only a minimal effect. At this point, the patient is likely to decompensate rapidly, and this is very difficult to reverse. Consequently, rapid diagnosis and transportation to the nearest hospital with obstetric surgical facilities (with a pre-alert en route) is essential to facilitate control of haemorrhage at the earliest possible time. Cannulation and intravenous fluids should only be initiated en route to hospital to avoid any delay on scene.

TOP TIP

Delaying on scene to start an intravenous infusion only allows further blood loss to occur and greatly increases the risk of irreversible decompensation.

TOP TIP

The treatment of obstetric haemorrhage is early surgery. This is best facilitated by short on-scene times and a pre-alert message on the way to the nearest hospital, preferably with obstetric theatres.

Uterus and genital tract

The uterus and genital tract enlarge during pregnancy and the blood supply increases to meet the energy requirements of the muscular uterus and the growing fetus. The high muscle tone in the uterus raises the risk of it tearing following trauma, and its excellent blood supply significantly increases the likelihood of major haemorrhage. Consideration must be given to those women who have had a previous caesarean section, as there is a two- to three-fold risk of uterine rupture during second and subsequent pregnancies (RCOG, 2015).

Gastrointestinal system

Although nausea and vomiting are common in early pregnancy, the presence of severe vomiting (hyperemesis gravidarum) can rapidly lead to dehydration, electrolyte imbalance and weight loss. It is a condition that affects around 1:100 pregnant women. This condition often requires fluid replacement and the use of antiemetics.

As described in the airway section, gastric tone and emptying rates are reduced in pregnancy, particularly during late pregnancy and even more so during labour. Although secretion of gastric acid is reduced in mid-pregnancy, this rises above normal levels at the end of the third trimester. The cardiac sphincter is relatively lax as a consequence of the effects of progesterone, and the gravid uterus compresses the stomach, potentially displacing its contents into the oesophagus. As a consequence of these changes, there is a greater risk of gastric reflux and aspiration, made worse by the increased acidity of stomach contents.

> **TOP TIP**
>
> **Failure to effectively secure the airway in unconscious obstetric patients is associated with an increased risk of aspiration pneumonia.**

Renal system

From the first trimester onwards, the kidneys and ureters become displaced as a result of compression by the enlarging uterus. These changes result in an increasing incidence of urinary tract infections, nephrolithiasis and pyelonephritis. Frequency of micturation, urgency and incontinence can also occur as the fetal head engages in the pelvis during the third trimester.

5.2 Relevant laboratory tests – differences in the 'normal range' in pregnancy

Table 5.1 shows the main differences in results between the pregnant and non-pregnant state (Heslehurst et al., 2007). When no difference occurs then the non-pregnant value is given. Table 5.2 provides a summary of the key points.

Table 5.1 Ranges of values for laboratory tests

Test	Non-pregnant	Pregnant/immediate postnatal	Reason
Full blood count			
Hb (g/l)	118–148	105–135	Haemodilution
WBC × 10^9 per litre	4–11	8–18	Due to increased neutrophil count
Platelets × 10^9 per litre	150–400	200–600	
MCV (fl)	77–98		
ESR (mm/h)	2–36		
CRP (mg/l)	<5		
Renal function			
Urea (mmol/l)	2.8–7.6	2.4–4.2	Increase in GFR Vasodilatation
Creatinine (micromol/l)	44–80	44–73	Lowest in mid-trimester
K (mmol/l)	3.5–5.2	3.2–4.6	
Na (mmol/l)	135–145	132–140	
Uric acid (mmol/l)	0.14–0.34	0.14–0.38	
Bilirubin (micromol/l)	0–17	3–16	

Important note: always refer to local reference values.

Some tests vary according to gestation in which case the range of values covers all stages.

Table 5.3 gives examples of blood results obtained in different clinical conditions (this is not an exhaustive list but contains some common or important examples).

Table 5.2 Summary of key points	
Lower in pregnancy	**Higher in pregnancy**
Haemoglobin	White cell count
Urea	Alkaline phosphate
Creatinine	pH
Sodium	PaO_2
Potassium	
Protein	
Bilirubin	
Bicarbonate	
$PaCO_2$	

Table 5.3 Interpretation of abnormal values		
Test	**High**	**Low**
Haemoglobin		Anaemia
		Sickle-cell disease
		Thalassaemia
White cell count	Infection	
Clotting factors (APTT, PT)		DIC
		Abruption
		Severe pre-eclampsia
Urea and creatinine	Renal failure	
	Dehydration	
	Pre-eclampsia	
Urate	Pre-eclampsia	
Liver function tests	Severe pre-eclampsia	
	HELLP	
	Cholestasis	
	Hepatitis (viral)	
	Acute fatty liver of pregnancy	
Platelets		Severe pre-eclampsia
		HELLP
		DIC
Glucose	Diabetes	Acute fatty liver of pregnancy

Summary of key points

- Early airway management is essential in any obtunded obstetric patient as changes to the gastrointestinal system increase the risk of aspiration
- Obstetric patients have little respiratory reserve
- Obstetric patients may initially compensate for blood loss due to their increased circulatory volume; however, this will be at the expense of the blood supply to the fetus
- Obstetric patients may suddenly decompensate rapidly following haemorrhage; this is often irreversible. Be aware of a rising pulse and respiratory rate
- Obstetric patients are at increased risk of postural hypotension and should be encouraged to change position slowly
- Never lie a patient who is >20 weeks' pregnant supine in order to avoid aortocaval compression, which can lead to maternal and fetal hypoxia
- Increased coagulation factors during pregnancy increase the risk of deep venous thrombosis/pulmonary embolism

CHAPTER 6
Structured approach to the obstetric patient

Learning outcomes

After reading this chapter, you will be able to:
- Describe the structured approach to assessing an obstetric patient
- Perform obstetric primary and secondary surveys
- Demonstrate the correct approach in taking an obstetric history
- Identify the key features of an obstetric history

6.1 Structured approach

A practitioner's approach to any clinical encounter should always be predictable and structured. This approach:

- Enables early and continual identification of life-threatening conditions
- Assists in a systematic and thorough assessment of the patient
- Minimises the possibility of missing signs, symptoms or conditions
- Promotes a professional attitude
- Protects against criticism or complaint

The structured approach to an obstetric patient augments the standard approach to increase awareness of the signs and symptoms likely to compromise the mother and/or the unborn baby. The responding practitioner carries out a quick scan of the scene and the patient as they approach. This is referred to as a 'global overview'. The standard ABCDE approach is maintained and extended to ABCDEFG. The 'F' refers to the fundus and the 'G' encourages the practitioner to 'get to the point quickly' in order to facilitate transfer for appropriate care. The right level of definitive care for an obstetric patient includes a properly equipped obstetric department, operating theatre or emergency department.

6.2 Obstetric primary survey

Global overview

The obstetric primary survey consists of the first 'hands-on' examination of the pregnant patient. In the pre-hospital environment, the responding practitioner needs to make an assessment of the situation as they approach the patient, before starting the primary survey (Figure 6.1). This global overview is a 'hands-off' process and starts to corral the practitioner's thoughts on the seriousness of the situation. During the global overview, the following should be considered:

Pre-Obstetric Emergency Training: A Practical Approach, Second Edition. Edited by Mark Woolcock.
© 2019 John Wiley & Sons Ltd. Published 2019 by John Wiley & Sons Ltd.

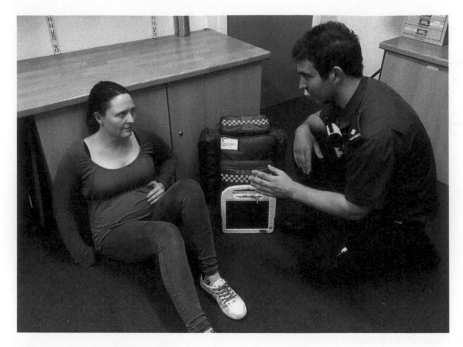

Figure 6.1 Obstetric primary survey – global overview

- Circulation/massive external haemorrhage – this is defined as catastrophic haemorrhage that is readily visible without the need to disturb the patient's clothing
- Airway – is the patient talking, making snoring or gurgling sounds, or not making any sounds at all?
- Breathing – is the patient speaking in whole sentences? Have they adopted a position that suggests respiratory compromise?
- Circulation – is the patient pale or flushed, or a normal colour?
- Disability – is the patient talking, moving or making sounds?
- Environment – is there blood on the floor or clothing of the patient? Has the baby been born yet? What position is the patient in? Is the home clean? Is it warm? Are there other children present?
- Fundus – does the patient look as if she is in the first, second or third trimester?
- Get to the point quickly – start the primary survey!

Primary survey

The obstetric primary survey consists of the first 'hands-on' examination of the pregnant patient. The aim of the primary survey is to rapidly identify life-threatening problems through a systematic and structured approach, and to manage each problem as it is encountered. It is important to reach an early determination of the priority for transportation. The primary survey should be modified in the presence of trauma – see Chapter 10 for details.

It is important to remember there are potentially two patients – neither the mother nor a newly born baby should be overlooked whilst assessing and caring for the other. Both may be at risk, or one may need more urgent attention than the other – it may not be possible to determine which until a primary survey has been completed on both patients. For the primary survey of newborn babies, see Chapter 14.

Circulation/massive external haemorrhage

- Is there a significant volume of blood visible without the need to disturb the patient's clothing?
  - On the floor?
  - Is the patient's clothing soaked?
  - Are there a number of blood-soaked pads?

TOP TIP

Massive external haemorrhage, although rare, MUST be managed immediately (if compressible) or the patient may exsanguinate before the primary survey is completed.

Airway

- Is the patient able to talk? *(yes would indicate the airway is clear)*
- Is the patient making unusual sounds? *(gurgling suggests fluid in the airway, snoring suggests tongue/swelling/foreign body obstruction)*
- Protect the cervical spine if significant injury is suspected
- If the patient is unresponsive, open and inspect the airway and consider suction or removal of any obstruction

> **TOP TIP**
>
> **If you identify an airway problem, manage this before moving on to the next stage of the primary survey.**
>
> **If you are unable to open an obstructed airway, apply additional advanced airway skills with the shortest possible delay: this may require rapid transportation to the nearest hospital (regardless of the availability of obstetric skills) or you may have a practitioner at scene with advanced airway management skills.**

Breathing

- Assess the presence, work and efficacy of breathing; acknowledge respiratory rate and effort
- Assess for the presence of cyanosis, tracheal deviation or neck vein distension
- If not breathing adequately, ventilate
- In alert and responding patients, obtain an oxygen saturation level and administer oxygen based on clinical findings
- Inspect and palpate for chest movement and symmetry
- Percuss for resonance, and auscultate for added sounds

> **TOP TIP**
>
> **Increased respiratory rates without increased work of breathing may indicate an attempt to compensate for a circulatory problem.**

> **TOP TIP**
>
> **Routinely administering oxygen to a 'well' patient during normal labour is neither helpful nor clinically indicated, and may alarm the patient unnecessarily.**

> **TOP TIP**
>
> **Patients with respiratory rates of less than 10 or greater than 29 may require ventilatory support as they could indicate inadequate minute volumes and respiratory distress.**

Circulation

- In an unresponsive patient, assess for signs of circulation
- In an alert and responding patient, assess the radial pulse rate and volume
- Assess skin colour and temperature
- Assess for bleeding – check underwear, pads, the surface the patient is sitting on, and briefly examine the introitus with the patient's consent and considering their privacy. Ask the patient about bleeding – if they have discarded pads, how saturated were they? How many pads have they used in what time period?
- Measure blood pressure
- Think 'BLOOD ON THE FLOOR AND FIVE MORE' (Box 6.1)

Box 6.1 'Blood on the floor and five more'

- BLOOD ON THE FLOOR – check for visible blood loss again and feel under any clothing or bed linen the patient is sitting or lying on, as this can absorb significant volumes of blood. Look at your gloved hands to see if they are stained with blood
- FIVE MORE (look and feel):
  1. Check the introitus for evidence of bleeding (soaked pads or underwear, wounds)
  2. Check the thoracic area for evidence of internal bleeding following trauma (tenderness, wounds, crepitus, patterning from clothes and seatbelts, discolouration)
  3. Check the abdominal area for evidence of internal bleeding (tenderness, guarding, firm woody uterus, wounds, patterning from clothes and seatbelts, discolouration)
  4. Check the pelvis for evidence of injury following trauma (consider mechanism – high speed impact with other significant injuries; complaint of hip or low back pain; bruising). NB do not compress or 'spring' the pelvis as this may dislodge clots
  5. Check the femurs for signs of fracture following trauma (swelling, tenderness, deformity, open fractures)

Figure 6.2 indicates how difficult it can be to estimate blood loss when encountered on different materials and surfaces.

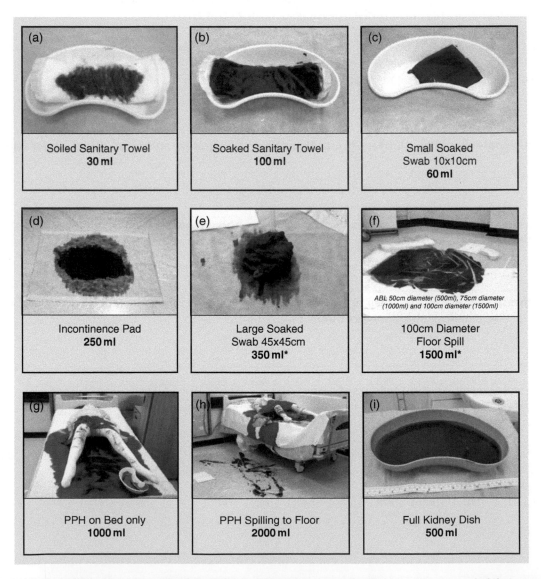

Figure 6.2 Estimating obstetric blood loss. *Multidisciplinary observations of estimated blood loss revealed that scenarios (e–f) are grossly underestimated (>30%). (Source: Bose P, Regan F, Paterson-Brown S. Improving the accuracy of estimated blood loss at obstetric haemorrhage using clinical reconstructions. BJOG, 18 July 2006. Reproduced with permission of John Wiley & Sons)

> **TOP TIP**
>
> **If this is an antepartum haemorrhage, the optimum treatment is surgery in an obstetric theatre. Do not delay transportation to gain vascular access; fluids (if indicated) should be started in the ambulance en route to the hospital.**
>
> **There is NO evidence that pre-hospital IV fluids saves lives. There is good evidence that short on-scene times and pre-alerting the hospital DO save lives.**

> **TOP TIP**
>
> **In a full-term patient in labour, any blood loss making a stain larger in diameter than a drink's coaster is cause for significant concern.**

Disability

- Perform an AVPU assessment of conscious level (is the patient **a**lert, responding only to **v**oice, responding only to **p**ain, or **u**nresponsive?)
- Assess patient's neurological status
- Assess the patient's position and note any abnormal posture (convulsing, abnormal flexion, abnormal extension)
- Assess pupil size and reaction

Expose/environment/evaluate

- If you have not already done so, briefly examine the introitus – is there any evidence of bleeding? Can you see a presenting part of the baby? Is there a prolapsed loop of cord? Have the waters broken? Does the perineum bulge with each contraction? If the baby has been delivered, is there a significant perineal tear? Can you see part of the uterus?
- Is the environment warm and discrete? Are the surroundings as clean as you can make them if you are going to deliver on site?
- Make an early evaluation about how time critical the patient's problem is. If the patient's status is time critical, decide immediately whether you need to transport the patient urgently to hospital, or whether it is more prudent to treat them at the scene – remember to call for skilled obstetric help if this is the case

> **TOP TIP**
>
> **Predicting the time of delivery is impossible, however it is not best practice to deliver a baby in the back of an ambulance: these have inadequate space, heating and lighting, and are unhygienic. Early planning to stay or transfer will help avoid 'mobile births'.**

Fundus

- Make a quick assessment of fundal height (Figure 6.3): a fundus at the level of the umbilicus equates to a gestation of approximately 20 weeks. By definition, a fundal height below the umbilicus suggests that if the fetus is delivered it is unlikely to survive

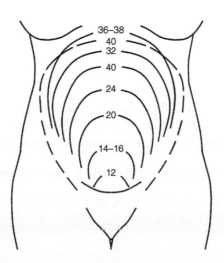

Figure 6.3 Fundal height estimation

Get to the point quickly

- Remember the aim is to identify time-critical problems as quickly as possible, to allow for rapid management and, if appropriate, transfer to a suitable obstetric facility for definitive care. These problems include:
  - Significant blood loss at any stage of pregnancy or in the postpartum period
  - Suspected abruption, placenta praevia or uterine rupture
  - Eclampsia or significant hypertension
  - Shoulder dystocia
  - Cord prolapse
  - Suspected amniotic fluid embolus
  - Retained placenta
  - Uterine inversion
  - Cervical shock
  - Refractory maternal cardiac arrest
  - Refractory neonatal cardiac arrest
  - Newborn with poor vital signs

Patients who have one or more of these problems are unlikely to be comprehensively managed outside of an obstetric facility.

If transport to hospital is possible, the care provided on scene should be restricted to that necessary to secure the patient's airway, ensure adequate ventilation and to control significant compressible haemorrhage.

TOP TIP: ASSESSING FUNDAL HEIGHT

To palpate the fundus, either use the ulnar aspect or a palm of one hand and feel for the upper aspect of the gravid uterus. A measure can then be taken from the fundus to the pubic symphysis. This distance in centimetres roughly corresponds to the weeks of gestation.

6.3 Positioning the patient

A responsive obstetric patient should be assisted into a position of comfort, which is most likely to be the semi-recumbent position (Figure 6.4).

In an unresponsive and noticeably pregnant woman, i.e. one with a significant intra-abdominal mass (usually by 20 weeks), it is important to obtain a left lateral tilt of the pelvis at the earliest opportunity to minimise the risk of aortocaval compression.

There is a range of opinion on the amount of left lateral tilt that should be achieved and maintained. Around 15 degrees is usually sufficient to reduce vena caval compression, and around 30 degrees to reduce aortal compression. However, the latter may be difficult to achieve.

In the absence of custom-made wedges, the unresponsive patient should be placed in a full left lateral position, or her uterus should be manually displaced. Where a patient requires full spinal immobilisation, it is important to ensure that the orthopaedic stretcher or rescue board is tilted to 15-30° to the left, with adequate strapping to secure the woman (Figure 6.5).

TOP TIP

1. **For a conscious woman who is unwell and is able to maintain her airway, adopting a comfortable semi-recumbent position is ideal.**
2. **If the woman is unconscious, e.g. in eclampsia, left lateral tilt or manual uterine displacement will relieve aortocaval pressure.**
3. **Any pregnant woman more than 20 weeks' pregnant, who is in cardiac arrest, should be managed supine with manual uterine displacement applied (this may be by a relative or a person instructed by the practitioner.**

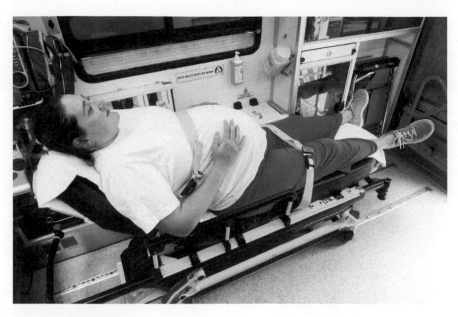

Figure 6.4 Patient in semi-recumbent position

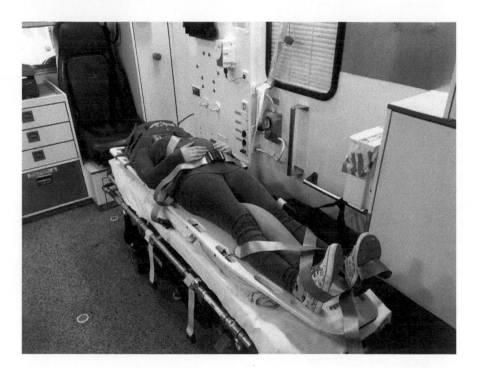

Figure 6.5 Patient on spinal board with left lateral tilt

6.4 Taking and evaluating an obstetric history

A robust obstetric history involves five areas of questioning. These are: (i) any past medical or surgical history; (ii) any medications or allergies; (iii) any past obstetric history; (iv) the history of the current pregnancy; and (v) the history of the current problem. It is essential to request and read the patient's hand-held maternity notes whenever possible, as these will provide key collateral information that the patient may omit to provide. It is also helpful to confirm:

- The patient's name
- Date of birth or age
- Which hospital the woman has booked for her care in pregnancy, and indeed IF she has booked. Remember it may be a concealed or phantom pregnancy
- Is the woman booked under consultant-led or midwife-led care (the latter will indicate that the mother is booked for low-risk antenatal care)?

It is essential to determine the gestation of pregnancy through the estimated date of delivery (EDD). This may be difficult to determine if the woman has not received any antenatal care or has not booked in. You may have to use the last menstrual period (LMP) (if known) as a marker.

Past medical and surgical history

- Is there a history of hypertension, thromboembolic disease, epilepsy, diabetes, asthma or other major medical conditions?
- What surgical procedures have occurred?
- When, where and why for all hospital admissions
- Any mental health history, including depression, self-harm, etc.
- Has any gynaecological surgery occurred (LLETZ (large loop excision of transformation zone), D&C (dilatation and curettage), etc.)?
- Any significant gynaecological history, treatment for infertility, treatment for urinary tract infections, pelvic inflammatory disease, etc.

Medications and allergies

- What medications are currently prescribed and how has the patient's compliance been?
- Which – if any – medications have been started in regard to pregnancy (such as folates, iron, antiemetics or antacids)?
- Have any over-the-counter (OTC) drugs been taken that the patient has sourced and started themselves?
- Any history or current use of recreational or illicit drugs (this is a leading cause of maternal death)
- Any allergies or sensitivities

Past obstetric history

- Gravidity: total number of pregnancies, including current one
- Parity: the total number of birth events resulting in a live birth (at any gestation) or a stillbirth (defined as a baby born dead after gestation of more than 24 weeks). Include any miscarriage or terminations (consideration needs to be paid to when, where and how this line of questioning is delivered)
- Have there been any ectopic pregnancies?
- Length of previous pregnancies
- Was labour induced or spontaneous?
- Mode of delivery in the past: normal vaginal delivery, assisted vaginal birth, operative vaginal delivery or caesarean section
- Were there any complications antenatally (e.g. haemorrhage, hyperemesis gravidarum, eclampsia, intrauterine growth restriction), during labour (e.g. premature birth, failure to progress, perineal tears, shoulder dystocia) or postnatally (e.g. postpartum haemorrhage, retained products of conception)?
- Weight of any previous babies

History of current pregnancy

- LMP or gestation
- How was the pregnancy confirmed (home testing kit, hCG blood test, ultrasound scan)?
- Any problems so far
- What scans have occurred so far (dating scan, anomaly scan)?
- Number of babies: singleton, twins or higher multiple
- Care booked with midwife, shared care or consultant-led care?
- Any concerns with the baby

> **TOP TIP**
>
> **In assisted conceptions, the given EDD is highly reliable, as it is based on the date of embryo transfer. With natural conceptions, an early ultrasound scan increases the reliability of EDD, as compared with the LMP alone.**

History of current problem

Questions should be aimed at clarifying the current problem. The following scheme helps capture significant problems:

Labour

- Number of contractions in 10-minute period
- How strong, how long do they last (seconds/minutes)?
- Feels like pushing
- Anything hanging between legs – for example a cord

Pain

- Type – constant, intermittent. Contractions – does the uterus go hard, coming and going, stabbing, ache?
- Severity – worst pain ever, score on a scale of 0–10
- Location:
  - Abdomen – over uterus, low down, under ribs, one side, back
  - Chest – central, one side, back
  - Head – frontal, unilateral
- Radiation – does the pain go anywhere else or does it stay in one place?
- Relieving and exacerbating factor – what, if anything, makes the pain worse or better?

Discharge

- Colour – clear or green, yellow, pink, red?
- Odour – odourless, offensive, smell of urine?
- Consistency – watery, thick, jelly-like, frothy?
- Quantity – gush, trickle, still draining?

Bleeding

- When did it start?
- Quantity: only on wiping after going to toilet, teaspoon, eggcup, soak pants/trousers, sanitary towel, bath towel, blood easily seen running down legs to toes?
- Still bleeding?
- Clots – are there any and if so how big?
- Is the blood mixed with mucus?

Seizures

- Previous history of seizures/epilepsy
- Any witnesses?
- Tonic-clonic movements – how long for?
- Associated incontinence, biting tongue/lips
- Postictal state

Fetal movements

- Is the baby moving normally?
- Is the baby moving less?
- When was the last time she felt the baby move?

Evaluating the history

- Assess the history for risk factors
- Assess symptom severity
- Attempt to make a diagnosis
- Use examination findings to confirm diagnosis (refer to subsequent chapters for guidance regarding risk factors and the significance of signs)

Box 6.2 gives some general hints.

Box 6.2 Key findings from history and examination

- Labour is established if there are three or more contractions in 10 minutes
- If there are more than five contractions in 10 minutes consider the diagnosis of abruption
- Rectal pressure may mean she is fully dilated or that the baby is coming down in the occipitoposterior (OP) position
- If there is severe pain with no fetal movement with or without bleeding – assume placental abruption until proven otherwise
- Hypertension increases the risk of abruption
- Bleeding that reaches the toes is significant
- Any bleeding with a low-lying placenta is significant
- Previous caesarean section increases the risk of uterine rupture
- Breech presentation and transverse lie have a higher chance of cord prolapse
- Previous preterm delivery increases the likelihood of another preterm delivery
- Twin pregnancies have an increased risk of all obstetric complications
- If there is a history of a seizure in the absence of a history of epilepsy – the woman should be considered to have had an eclamptic fit until proven otherwise (NB blood pressure may not be elevated at the time of the fit)
- Dead babies can 'move' like any immobile object in a pool of fluid (an external movement can cause the baby to knock against the uterine wall and this can be interpreted as a movement)

TOP TIP

Do not confuse gravidity with parity:

- **Gravidity = total number of pregnancies, including current one**
- **Parity = total number of birth events resulting in a live birth (at any gestation) or a stillbirth (defined as a baby born dead after gestation of more than 24 weeks). A twin delivery is recorded as a single birth event for gravidity**

6.5 Obstetric secondary survey

The obstetric secondary survey should only be undertaken when time-critical factors identified during the primary survey have been addressed and transportation to definitive care has commenced (if this is possible). In some cases it will not be possible or appropriate to undertake a secondary survey in the pre-hospital phase of care.

Secondary survey

Perform an examination:

- Review the airway patency
- Review the breathing: respiratory rate and quality
- Review the circulation: pulse rate and quality
- Assess again for blood loss:
  - Look to see how much, note any soaked garments or bed linen. (If yes, why are you doing a secondary survey?)
    - Beware of blood loss down to the toes. (If yes, why are you doing a secondary survey?)
    - Ask to see any visible active vaginal bleeding by vulval inspection.
    - Is it fresh red bleeding or watery?
    - Are there any clots?
  - Check the blood pressure
- Review disability – assess Glasgow Coma Scale (GCS) score, pupils, posture and seizures
- Review your evaluation – is this still a non-time-critical patient?

- If time and the patient's condition permit, undertake a basic obstetric examination:
  - Inspect the abdomen for:
    - abdominal scars
    - cutaneous signs (striae gravidarum, linea nigra)
    - oedema
    - fetal movements
  - Palpate the abdomen for:
    - tenderness
    - rigidity
    - uterine contractions
    - fundal height
    - lie/presentation/position
    - fetal movements
  - Auscultate the abdomen for:
    - fetal heart sounds if proficient in this technique
- Attempt to assess the fetal lie and presentation, and feel for the head in a pregnancy of >32 weeks' gestation
- If the woman is contracting and is in apparent labour, palpate the contractions for strength and frequency
- A vulval inspection will be necessary if the woman is feeling the urge to push (or if there has been any concern about vaginal bleeding)
- Look for visible signs of the second stage of labour such as:
  - Anal dilatation
  - Presence of the head (or other presenting part) at the introitus
  - Look for the signs of a cord prolapse, particularly if the woman has had a sudden spontaneous rupture of her membranes
- If there has been a spontaneous rupture of membranes, assess the colour of the liquor. Is it:
  - Clear?
  - Blood stained?
  - Meconium stained?
  - Turbid or offensive?

If a vulval inspection is necessary, remember the following:

- **ALWAYS** ask for the woman's consent to perform this inspection, and explain why you need to do it. You should document that you have obtained consent in the notes
- Explain to the partner or relative accompanying the woman
- Have someone with you if possible (ideally another healthcare practitioner)
- Maintain the woman's dignity. Cover her up immediately following the examination
- Acknowledge cultural variations, as this forms part of the consent process
- Respect the woman's right to refuse
- You should request a urine sample from all stable and non-time-critical patients for bedside urinalysis
- Always obtain at least one set of vital observations, which should include conscious level, pulse rate, blood pressure, respiratory rate, oxygen saturation, temperature and blood glucose level

---

TOP TIP: ASSESSING THE FETAL LIE

This is the position of the fetal long axis in relation to the mother. In a pregnancy of >32 weeks, palpate the abdomen to find the baby's back and limbs. The limbs will feel irregular and lack continuity in shape, however the back will be felt as a regular curve. The lie should be described as longitudinal, transverse or oblique:

- **A longitudinal lie is where the fetal spine is in line (parallel) with the mother's spine**
- **A transverse lie is where the fetal spine is at 90 degrees (perpendicular) to the mother**
- **An oblique lie is where the fetal spine is neither longitudinal nor transverse**

There is a range of opinion on the value of palpating the abdomen or assessing fetal lie when making a decision to transport. The baby will not deliver if in a transverse or oblique lie. Recognition of the presenting part at the introitus (i.e. feet, buttocks or hand/arm) is a better indication.

Lie can be difficult to palpate unless specifically trained, especially in women with a raised body mass index (BMI).

Guidance on performing internal vaginal examinations

Internal vaginal examination should not be routinely performed by non-obstetric practitioners but reserved for critical and clinically indicated situations, and in relation to obstetric emergencies such as delivery of the aftercoming head in a breech presentation, or prolapsed cord.

Measuring blood pressure

The 2006–08 UK Confidential Enquiry into Maternal Deaths report (CMACE, 2011) provided resounding evidence on how the accuracy of blood pressure (BP) measurement impacted on maternal and perinatal clinical outcomes.

Whether assessing for hypertension or managing a patient who is haemorrhaging or who has a pregnancy-related sepsis, the reliance on accurate BP measurement is profound.

The National Institute for Health and Care Excellence (NICE) *Antenatal Care* guidance (NICE, 2008) indicates routine BP measurement, and emphasises the use of a correctly sized cuff, initially inflating the cuff 20–30 mmHg above a palpable systolic BP and deflating at 2 mmHg per second.

The NICE guideline on antenatal care provides clear direction and recommends that Korotkoff phase V is more reflective of intra-arterial pressure and should be used (see Chapter 5).

The NICE guidelines on hypertension (NICE, 2010) in pregnancy make the following definitions:

- **Mild hypertension**: diastolic BP 90–99 mmHg and/or systolic BP 140–149 mmHg
- **Moderate hypertension**: diastolic BP 100–109 mmHg and/or systolic BP 150–159 mmHg
- **Severe hypertension**: diastolic BP >110 mmHg and/or systolic BP >160 mmHg

There are many ways of checking a pregnant woman's blood pressure. The manual aneroid devices form an integral part of most practitioners' response or crash equipment. However, these devices are user dependent and need regular calibration. Automated devices overcome these drawbacks, but there has been concern that automated devices tend to underestimate BP in women with pre-eclampsia due to specific pathological changes that occur in the pregnant woman. Thus, as long as aneroid devices are regularly calibrated and maintained, and the user's technique is robust, the measurement is viewed as reliable (Nathan et al., 2015).

A systolic BP of 100 mmHg is not uncommon in healthy pregnant women. However, as a guide, a systolic BP of less than 90 mmHg should be acknowledged as indicative of shock if other signs are present. At the other end of the scale, a systolic BP of 160 mmHg or over requires urgent medical assessment and treatment, as recommended within the CEMACH (2007a) report.

Always read the patient hand-held records to assess the trend in the woman's blood pressure, and assess for other clinical signs and symptoms for underlying disease or illness.

Fetal assessment

This is limited in the pre-obstetric setting, particularly in emergency situations.

Although fetal heart sounds can be heard with a standard stethoscope, they may be difficult to hear, and are not an assurance of fetal well-being. In cases of placental abruption, fetal heart sounds may be muffled or difficult to hear if there is concealed bleeding within the uterus. Transfer should not be delayed by attempting to auscultate the fetal heart.

Using a standard stethoscope, start listening for the heartbeat near the place you believe the fetal heart to be. It may be necessary to listen in many places on the mother's abdomen before locating the place where the heartbeat is clearest and loudest. A heartbeat that is loudest below the mother's umbilicus suggests the baby is probably in a cephalic presentation, while a heartbeat that is loudest above the umbilicus may suggest the baby is in a breech presentation.

Asking the mother about fetal movements is one way of attempting to determine fetal well-being. However, the absence of movements does not indicate a poor outcome. The fetus does not move all of the time and may be in a sleep cycle. The mother may not always feel fetal movements if she is contracting frequently.

Assessing the colour of the liquor if the membranes have ruptured is another way to assess fetal well-being. If fresh meconium is present in the liquor it will be a yellowy-green colour with particulate matter present. The presence of fresh meconium or heavy blood staining gives cause for concern and alerts the need for appropriate fetal monitoring when the woman is transferred into the hospital setting.

TOP TIP

Do not delay the transportation of the mother through attempting to determine fetal well-being.

6.6 Handover of the obstetric patient

A clinical handover to another healthcare practitioner is a crucial point in the management of any patient. If this is not performed correctly, important information may be missed, resulting in incorrect or delayed diagnoses and treatment.

A verbal handover should be structured to avoid missing any vital information, succinct to maintain attention and precise to minimise delay in the clinical takeover. Remember that a preliminary stage of the handover process to a hospital may be the pre-alert message and this can use the same structure. ATMISTER is commonly used between pre-hospital practitioners and emergency department staff, and provides the basis for a concise and informative pre-alert message.

A – Age
T – Time of incident (trauma) / Time of onset (medical)
M – Mechanism of injury (trauma) / Medical complaint/history (medical)
I – Injuries (trauma) / Investigations (medical)
S – vital Signs (first set and significant changes)
T – Treatment
E – Estimated time of arrival (ETA)
R – Requirements, e.g. bloods, specialist services, tiered response, ambulance call sign

On arriving at hospital a verbal handover should occur. It is acceptable to use ATMISTER as the basis for this information exchange – particularly in the emergency department. Some practitioners find a more comprehensive clinical handover is required when liaising with non-emergency department staff or carrying out a telephone referral. The SBAR (situation, background, assessment and recommendation) tool was specifically developed for use in healthcare (Leonard et al., 2006), and is believed to improve the efficiency of inter-professional communication. See Chapter 4 for more information on communicating with other healthcare professionals. The elements of a SBAR clinical handover are:

- **Situation**: the practitioner introduces the patient by name, states their age and gestational state and describes their specific situation or condition
- **Background**: a précis of the patient's medical history is required, as well as their previous obstetric history. It is essential to provide an accurate summary of the current pregnancy
- **Assessment**: this involves a critical assessment of the situation, a clinical impression and a detailed expression of concerns
- **Recommendation**: this may be as pointed as 'so that is why we are here' but in general terms should reflect why the admission is necessary. It may involve a request to accept a referral, a request for expert advice or a conversation to devise a management plan

Following verbal handover of the patient, all findings and treatment provided must be recorded either in writing or electronically, and where possible a copy provided for the attention of the receiving staff and for incorporating into the patient's hospital notes. If the patient is not hospitalised, the hand-held record should be updated and, where possible, a copy of their written or printed notes included. It is entirely acceptable to complete the patient record after the handover, particularly when managing a clinically unstable patient. The most important factor is not when the notes were written, but what was recorded. Always strive to maintain the highest level of clinical documentation.

Summary of key points

- Specific attention to minimising delays on scene is the preferred method of dealing with obstetric emergencies
- The primary obstetric survey should be preceded by a global overview
- The primary obstetric survey aims to identify time-critical problems as rapidly as possible. It is similar to any primary survey but includes an assessment of fundal height and places emphasis on the identification of urgent obstetric problems (remember ABCDEFG)
- When examining for haemorrhage, think 'BLOOD ON THE FLOOR AND FIVE MORE'
- In time-critical patients where transportation to hospital is possible, appropriate treatment on scene should be restricted to securing the airway, maintaining adequate ventilation and control of significant haemorrhage
- Severe pain with no fetal movement with or without visible bleeding should be considered as placental abruption until proven otherwise
- Bleeding that reaches the toes is significant
- Any bleeding with a low-lying placenta is significant
- Labour is established if there are three or more contractions in 10 minutes
- Rectal pressure may mean the pregnant woman is fully dilated or that the baby is coming down in the OP position
- Previous caesarean section increases the risk of uterine rupture
- Hypertension increases the risk of abruption
- If there are more than five contractions in 10 minutes consider the diagnosis of abruption
- Breech presentation and transverse lie have a higher chance of cord prolapse
- Previous preterm delivery increases the likelihood of another preterm delivery
- Twin pregnancies have an increased risk of all obstetric complications
- If there is a history of a seizure in the absence of a history of epilepsy, then the woman should be considered to have had an eclamptic fit until proven otherwise (NB blood pressure may not be elevated at the time of the fit)
- Dead babies can 'move' like any immobile object in a pool of fluid (an external movement can cause the baby to knock against the uterine wall and this can be interpreted as a movement)
- Do not delay the transportation of the mother by attempting to determine fetal well-being
- If transfer has commenced and delivery is imminent, divert to the nearest unit
- A pre-alert message should always be provided when transferring an obstetric emergency into hospital
- A careful clinical handover is essential; the use of ATMISTER or SBAR facilitates a structure to this conversation
- Ensure your clinical documentation is accurate, comprehensive and complete

CHAPTER 7
Collapse, cardiac arrest and shock in pregnancy

Learning outcomes

After reading this chapter, you will be able to:
- Describe the management of collapse and cardiac arrest in pregnancy
- Define the terms resuscitative hysterotomy (RH)/perimortem caesarean section (PMCS)
- Explain the situations when RH/PMCS should be considered
- Describe the management of shock in pregnancy

This chapter addresses the aetiology, identification and treatment of collapse and cardiac arrest, and shock during pregnancy. As the management of adult cardiac arrest is well documented in the Resuscitation Council (UK) guidelines, which are regularly updated, this chapter discusses only those differences specific to obstetric patients.

7.1 Cardiac arrest in pregnancy

Incidence

Cardiac arrest in pregnancy is rare, with maternal mortality rates varying by age, socioeconomic status and ethnic background. The higher rates are seen amongst older women, some ethnic minority groups and those living in the most deprived areas of the UK (MBRRACE-UK, 2015a).

Principles of resuscitation during pregnancy

The principles of resuscitation for the pregnant woman are similar to those of any adult cardiac arrest patient. Due to the physiological changes, after 20 weeks of pregnancy, some modifications to standard adult cardiac arrest algorithms are required to improve the efficiency of resuscitation.

Although the fetus can tolerate quite significant levels of hypoxia, it is still reliant on the mother's body for delivery of oxygenated blood. Consequently, resuscitation of the mother should always be initiated immediately, even if her injuries appear to be unsurvivable, and resuscitation should not be terminated in the pre-hospital setting. This approach will maximise the chances of both maternal and fetal survival.

The following section provides a summary of the main physiological changes that will require the pre-hospital practitioner to modify their approach:

Pre-Obstetric Emergency Training: A Practical Approach, Second Edition. Edited by Mark Woolcock.
© 2019 John Wiley & Sons Ltd. Published 2019 by John Wiley & Sons Ltd.

Airway

The mucosal lining of the upper airways become oedematous and slightly swollen due to hormonal changes of pregnancy. Airway insertion, specifically the nasopharyngeal airway, is associated with an increased risk of failure or minor trauma compared with the non-pregnant patient. In general, airways with a smaller internal diameter should be selected, and nasopharyngeal airways avoided (Battaloglu and Porter, 2016).

Particularly during the late stages of pregnancy, the gastro-oesophageal sphincter becomes lax, gastric emptying is delayed, gastric pressure rises and gastric fluids become more acidic, representing a significantly increased risk of regurgitation and aspiration pneumonia. Consequently, rapid escalation of airway interventions to insertion of a cuffed endotracheal (ET) tube is essential. Whilst this is the gold standard in airway management, if unavailable or an attempt fails, a supraglottic airway device such as an i-gel® will allow effective oxygenation but not protection from aspiration.

Breathing

It is estimated that the relaxed diaphragm will be elevated by the gravid uterus by up to 4 cm in the third trimester. The decreased compliance of the chest wall and splinting of the lungs by the diaphragm makes lung expansion much more difficult to achieve and requires higher pressures to facilitate, again potentially increasing the risk of gastric distension, regurgitation and aspiration. The added weight of engorged breasts may also contribute to reducing chest wall movement. Consequently, the mother's functional residual capacity will be reduced and the requirement of good bag–valve–mask (BVM) technique is paramount. The sizing of the face mask will remain unchanged.

Circulation

Due to the risk of aortocaval compression, a collapsed patient must be positioned in a left lateral tilt of between 15° and 30° or with the uterus manually displaced. However, when faced with a patient in cardiac arrest, the ability to deliver effective chest compressions is compromised when the patient is tilted and this will adversely affect the efficacy of any resuscitation attempt. Manual uterine displacement is now the recommended technique to overcome this. In addition to enabling effective chest compressions, manual uterine displacement enables easier access for airway management, bilateral vascular access and defibrillation.

Failure to reduce the risk of aortocaval compression will mean that oxygenated blood cannot be circulated to the mother or fetus. Occasionally, repositioning the uterus relative to the major blood vessels may reveal a profound syncope induced by aortocaval compression that has been misdiagnosed as a cardiac arrest.

> **TOP TIP**
>
> **Do not withhold resuscitation or terminate maternal resuscitation attempts in the pre-hospital setting as this may compromise the chances of maternal and fetal survival.**

Pre-hospital management

Patient positioning

Manual uterine displacement can be performed from the left of the patient (Figure 7.1) where the practitioner 'cups' and 'lifts' the uterus upwards and to the left off the maternal vessels. If the patient is loaded into an ambulance head first, manual uterine displacement can also be achieved from the right of the patient (Figure 7.2), where the uterus is pushed upwards and to the left. Care must be taken not to inadvertently push down, which would increase the amount of inferior vena cava compression and cancel any potential benefit.

Lateral tilt can be achieved by using an improvised wedge under the patient or by placing the patient on an immobilisation device before tilting (see Chapter 6). It is also a technique that can be used when fewer team members are present, for instance when transferring a patient in the ambulance with only one clinician in the saloon.

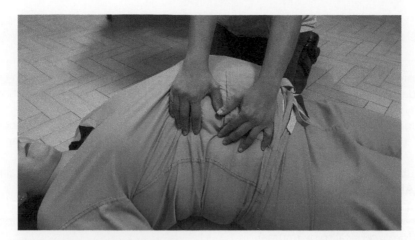

Figure 7.1 Manual uterine displacement ('cupping' technique)

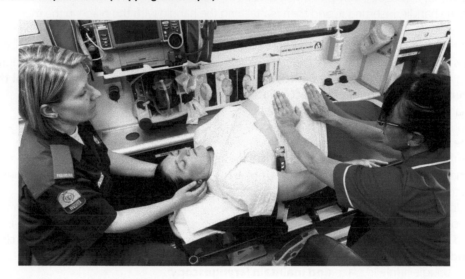

Figure 7.2 Manual uterine displacement (push technique)

Airway

The sizing and insertion of an oropharyngeal airway and supraglottic airway (SGA) device are unaltered. Care should be taken when inserting a nasopharyngeal airway due to the increased friability of the upper airway mucosa. With regard to selecting an ET tube it is recommended that the size should start at 7.0 and proceed to smaller tube selection if needed (size 6.0 and 5.0) as there is an association between larger tubes and glottic and tracheal damage in women (MBRRACE-UK, 2017).

Intubation of the trachea during the late stages of pregnancy can also be particularly challenging, due to:

- Presence of full dentition
- Short obese (oedematous) neck
- Engorged breasts
- Oedema and swelling of the upper airway
- Risk of regurgitation during intubation

Any strategy for the intubation of patients in the late stages of pregnancy must have the aim of minimising the time from commencing laryngoscopy to inflation of the tracheal tube cuff to reduce the risk of aspiration. All such interventions are, therefore, 'crash' intubations (Box 7.1). Additionally, any practitioner attempting to secure the airway must have a 'failed intubation' plan that should include the availability of a SGA device, such as the i-gel® or laryngeal mask airway (LMA).

TOP TIP

The choice of tracheal tube for pregnant women should start at size 7.0 and proceed to smaller tube selection if needed (size 6.0 and 5.0).

Box 7.1 Obstetric intubation strategy

1. Remember to proceed with left lateral tilt or manual uterine displacement.
2. Because of the pre-existing risk of regurgitation being exacerbated by ventilation using non-cuffed airway devices, minimise the tidal volume of ventilation via BVM and move as quickly as possible to intubation (do not waste time attempting to hyperventilate the patient).
3. Have suction running with the tip placed under the patient's shoulder; use wide-bore tubing, not an ET catheter.
4. Prepare the ET tube for a crash intubation: cut to length, and with a syringe, catheter mount and tube-tie pre-attached.
5. Prepare an ET tube introducer (bougie) for use, curving the bougie and ensuring the distal tip is formed into a J (coudé) shape. **Always use a bougie in the pre-hospital setting**.
6. Consider using a number 4 laryngoscope blade.
7. Use at least one pillow or equivalent to place the patient's head in the 'sniffing the morning air' position (unless there is a suspicion of cervical spine trauma).
8. Insertion of the laryngoscope may prove very difficult in obstetric patients. This may be overcome by removing the blade from the handle, inserting it, and then reattaching the handle with the blade in the mouth.
9. Since there is a high risk of regurgitation, an assistant should apply Sellick's manoeuvre. This differs from cricothyroid pressure in that one hand must be placed under the neck whilst the other manoeuvres the cricoid cartilage. This action helps to compress the oesophagus to minimise the risk of regurgitation, and has the additional benefit of bringing an anterior glottis into view. **Sellick's manoeuvre must not be discontinued until the ET tube has been correctly positioned and the cuff inflated**.
10. Perform a laryngoscopy, obtaining the best possible view of the glottic opening:
    a. You should always be able to view the tip of the epiglottis and, ideally, the arytenoid cartilages.
    b. Advance the bougie in the midline, continually observing its distal tip, with the concavity facing anteriorly.
    c. Visualise the tip of the bougie passing posterior to the epiglottis and (where possible) anterior to the arytenoid cartilages.
    d. Once the tip of the bougie has passed the epiglottis, continue to advance it in the midline so that it passes behind the epiglottis but in an anterior direction.
    e. As the tip of the bougie enters the glottic opening you will either feel 'clicks' as it passes over the tracheal rings or the tip will arrest against the wall of the airways ('hold-up'). This suggests correct insertion, although cannot be relied upon to indicate correct positioning with 100% accuracy. **However, failure to elicit clicks or hold-up is indicative of oesophageal placement**.
    f. Hold the bougie firmly in place **and maintain laryngoscopy**:
        i.   instruct a colleague to pass the ET tube over the proximal end of the bougie
        ii. as the proximal tip of the bougie is re-exposed, the assistant should carefully grasp it, assuming control of the bougie and passing control of the ET tube to the intubator
        iii. the ET tube should then be carefully advanced ('rail-roaded') along the bougie and hence through the glottic opening, taking care to avoid movement of the bougie
        iv. successful **intubation may be considerably enhanced by rotating the ET tube 90° anticlockwise, so that the bevel faces posteriorly**; in so doing the bougie will also rotate along the same plane but should not be allowed to move up or down the trachea
    g. Once the ET tube is fully in place, hold it securely as your colleague withdraws the bougie.
    h. Withdraw the laryngoscope.
11. Inflate the cuff without delay.
12. Verify correct positioning of the ET tube using auscultation of the lung fields and epigastrium and observing for chest wall movement. Do not just rely on visualising the tube passing through the cords.
13. Use a device or cord to secure the tube into place. The tip of the ET tube can move up to 6.0 cm once placed and this is certainly sufficient to dislodge it from the trachea. Record the figure on the side of the tube that is in line with the teeth.
14. Confirm tube placement using continuous quantitative waveform end-tidal CO_2 monitoring.
15. Position an appropriately sized oropharyngeal airway alongside the ET tube to serve as a bite block should the patient's level of consciousness change (unless the ET securing device has an integral bite block).
16. Each intubation attempt must take no more than 30 seconds from the point at which the last inflation was given to the time at which the first inflation is delivered via the tracheal tube. After 20 seconds has expired, if the tracheal tube has not been passed through the vocal cords, abandon the procedure and commence the failed intubation plan, which should include the use of a supraglottic airway device and careful monitoring for evidence of regurgitation. If ventilation is not possible move to surgical cricothyroidotomy.

Tracheal intubation with a cuffed tube is the gold standard of airway management, and this is particularly true in the obstetric patient due to the increased risk of regurgitation and aspiration of highly acidic stomach contents. However, it is a challenging procedure, particularly in third trimester patients and particularly if intubation skills are seldom practiced. Consequently, if it proves impossible to perform, alternative interventions must be considered.

Supraglottic airway devices

Insertion of an SGA device is performed without the need to visualise the glottis and it requires less skill to use than a tracheal tube. It is considered to be safer and more effective than naso- or oropharyngeal airways, producing less gastric distension during positive pressure ventilation and reducing the probability of regurgitation. However, if regurgitation does occur, a standard SGA is less effective than a tracheal tube at preventing aspiration. Further, the seal at the glottic opening is relatively weak and permits only low pressures to be used during ventilation. This can be a particular problem in late pregnancy as the chest wall is less compliant than normal and the lungs are splinted by the high diaphragm. Consequently, the SGA should only be used in obstetric patients if intubation skills are not available or intubation attempts have failed.

Surgical airway/cricothyroidotomy

Cricothyroidotomy is a technique of last resort in the pre-hospital environment. The procedure is basic in principle but often difficult when in clinical context. In particular, identification of the cricothyroid membrane can be challenging (Aslani et al., 2012).

An incision made vertically over the midline of the neck at the level of the cricothyroid cartilage increases the accuracy of locating the cricothyroid membrane and avoids incorrect tube placement. As with non-obstetric patients, the use of needle cricothyroidotomy provides an unsatisfactory method of oxygenation and is only recommended as a technique of extremis.

Breathing

Due to the increased metabolic requirement in pregnancy, the highest possible concentration of oxygen should be administered during ventilation, using an appropriate reservoir bag or automatic ventilator. To avoid cerebral vasoconstriction or vasodilatation in the mother and fetus, normocapnoea must be maintained and this is best facilitated by using an automatic ventilator in conjunction with waveform end-tidal CO_2 monitoring to set an appropriate rate and tidal volume.

Circulation

Chest compressions administered to a supine patient from 20 weeks of pregnancy onwards are unlikely to result in an adequate cardiac output due to the effects of aortocaval compression. As a brief intervention until help is available, a first responding clinician can position him- or herself to perform chest compressions with their knees under the patient's right posterior chest wall. The aim is to tilt the patient to the left to reposition the uterus.

As soon as possible (and as one of the first interventions to be performed when help arrives), this can be replaced with manual uterine displacement.

TOP TIP

Chest compressions administered to a supine patient after 20 weeks of pregnancy are unlikely to result in an adequate cardiac output unless the uterus is manually displaced to the left, or the patient is tilted on a firm surface.

7.2 Management of cardiac arrest

In general, the procedures and advanced life support protocols for managing cardiac arrest are the same for the obstetric patient as they are for any adult (Figure 7.3) although some modifications are recommended. Ventilation to compression ratios are the same as for any adult patient, although the hand placement for delivering a chest compression in a patient with advanced pregnancy (>28 weeks) may need to be 2–3 cm slightly higher up the sternum (RCUK, 2015). There is no evidence that transthoracic impedance is altered during pregnancy, thus energy levels remain unaltered. In patients with large breasts who are placed in the left lateral tilt position, attaching the defibrillation pad may be difficult, thus the anteroposterior or bi-axillary positions are acceptable (RCUK, 2015).

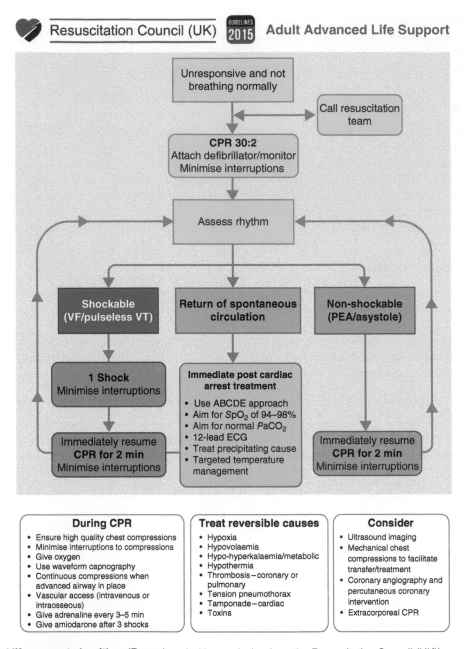

Figure 7.3 Advanced life support algorithm. (Reproduced with permission from the Resuscitation Council (UK))

If cardiac arrest is refractory to the completion of a second loop of 2 minutes of 30:2 cardiopulmonary resuscitation (CPR), the patient should be transported immediately with ongoing CPR to the nearest emergency department to enable RH/PMCS. CPR should *not* be terminated in the pre-hospital setting, even if the prognosis for the mother is poor. Any delays or pauses in CPR will significantly reduce the probability of survival of both the mother and the fetus.

> **TOP TIP**
>
> **The most common presenting cardiac arrest rhythm in pregnancy is pulseless electrical activity (PEA).**

As with victims of trauma, the treatment of cardiac arrest secondary to haemorrhage requires rapid surgical intervention in the obstetric patient, as the gravid uterus will compromise aortocaval blood flow. Indeed, if any pregnant woman of more than 20 weeks' gestation fails to respond to 4 minutes of active CPR, the aim is to perform RH/PMCS as soon as possible. Consequently, in all such cases, the patient should be rapidly transferred to an ambulance and positioned on stretcher with manual uterine displacement or applying 15–30° left lateral tilt. Their airway should be secured and urgent transport initiated, with a complete focus on minimising interruptions to chest compressions and ongoing CPR. The woman should be taken to the nearest emergency department with senior obstetric staff available on site. Consideration should be given to the reversible causes of cardiac arrest although there should be no delay on scene to cannulate the patient: rather this should be performed en route to hospital if enough rescuers are present. Crystalloids given in 250 ml aliquots should be administered. Consider the use of oxytocic drugs to correct uterine atony in postpartum haemorrhage (PPH) or the use of tranexamic acid in trauma.

> **TOP TIP**
>
> **Always pre-alert the receiving hospital if you are en route with a seriously ill or injured patient: ideally, speak directly to the senior obstetrician on call.**

> **TOP TIP**
>
> **Remaining on scene after more than 4 minutes of active CPR with no response will dramatically reduce the probability of survival for a mother and fetus after 20 weeks of pregnancy.**

7.3 Resuscitative hysterotomy/perimortem caesarean section

Definition

RH/PMCS is a modified type of caesarean section used after 20 weeks' gestation in cases of maternal cardiopulmonary arrest, when there has been no response to 4 minutes of active CPR. Both terms are used interchangeably and can be used singularly to indicate the same concept. The prime aim is to facilitate maternal resuscitation and maximise the chance of maternal survival. Although fetal survival is possible, this is not the prime aim of the procedure. RH/PMCS would still be considered for maternal reasons, even if the fetus was known to have died. The nearer to term that the incident has occurred, the better the chance of fetal survival. It is likely that at any gestation beyond 24 weeks (5–6 months), RH/PMCS would be performed to save both the mother's and infant's lives. Between 20 and 23 weeks it would be performed with the intention of saving the mother's life, as infant survival at this gestational age is unlikely. The procedure would not be indicated if the pregnancy was assessed as being less than 20 weeks as the gravid uterus would be unlikely to cause significant aortocaval compression.

All causes of maternal collapse may lead to cardiopulmonary arrest. One of the most common is major obstetric haemorrhage. Whatever the cause, active CPR with manual uterine displacement or left lateral tilt of 15–30° must be commenced and maintained until the patient is resuscitated or until arrival in the hospital setting. There is no place for pausing or ceasing active CPR as this will compromise the chances of maternal and fetal survival.

There is little published evidence to base practice on. However, physiology would suggest that RH/PMCS should be commenced after 4 minutes of active CPR if there is no maternal response. Ideally, it should be accomplished within 5 minutes of the onset of the arrest. Both maternal and fetal survival are maximised if these times can be accomplished. In one systematic review of 38 RH/PMCS cases in hospital, 34 infants and 13 mothers survived at discharge (ERC, 2015). Obviously with an arrest in the pre-hospital setting, outcomes may be less successful. However, there are reported cases of intact fetal survival when RH/PMCS has been started more than 20 minutes after the arrest. Although maternal outcome is extremely poor with delayed RH/PMCS, the fetal data should encourage maintenance of CPR throughout transfer. The transfer should also be undertaken as rapidly as possible, whilst ensuring high-quality, minimally interrupted chest compressions.

> **TOP TIP**
>
> **Rapid transfer to hospital with continuous CPR is recommended in cases of maternal cardiac arrest after 20 weeks' gestation.**

> **TOP TIP**
>
> **Perform RH/PMCS after 4 minutes after the cardiac arrest if resuscitation has failed to achieve a return of spontaneous circulation (ROSC) *and if appropriate facilities are available.***

Risk factors

- Any cause of maternal collapse resulting in cardiopulmonary arrest
- Obesity is a particular risk factor implicated in many causes of maternal collapse

Diagnosis

Use standard assessment techniques to diagnose maternal cardiac arrest and institute active CPR. RH/PMCS should be considered for all causes of cardiac arrest in pregnancy assessed to be more than 20 weeks, when active CPR has not led to signs of recovery within 4 minutes. An awareness of this timescale will encourage rapid transfer from the pre-hospital setting.

Pre-hospital management

1. Institute active CPR with manual uterine displacement or 15–30° of left lateral tilt.
2. Transfer to the nearest emergency department, preferably to a hospital with senior obstetric staff on site.
3. Provide a pre-alert – remember to ask for a senior obstetrician to be present on arrival.
4. Continue active CPR, minimising any pauses during transfer.
5. If vascular access has not been secured consider gaining access during transfer.

The steps in RH/PMCS are included as additional information in Box 7.2. The surgical technique for undertaking RH/PMCS requires little in the way of formal instrumentation. The most important issue is making the decision to proceed.

Box 7.2 Steps in RH/PMCS

This should be carried out by an appropriately qualified clinician AT HOSPITAL, in the emergency department or in the delivery suite, not in theatre, as this will save precious time.

1. Make the decision to proceed to RH/PMCS – and continue active CPR throughout the operation, until return of circulation.
2. Prepare for possible neonatal resuscitation.
3. Wear sterile gloves and apply basic skin preparation.
4. Rapid entry – use an appropriate incision in the abdominal wall and uterus.
5. Deliver the baby – hand over for assessment and possible resuscitation.
6. Leave the placenta in place – bleeding is minimal because of cardiac arrest.
7. Cardiac massage via the diaphragm may be considered with the abdomen open.
8. If resuscitation is successful, the anaesthetist will administer general anaesthesia.
9. Deliver the placenta and close the uterus and abdominal wall.
10. The patient must be transferred to theatre once return of circulation occurs.

7.4 Shock in pregnancy

Definition

Shock can be defined as a failure of perfusion of the tissues with oxygenated blood. This may be due to loss of circulating fluid volume due to haemorrhage (hypovolaemic shock), movement of circulating fluid volume into the interstitial spaces due to increased capillary permeability (septic shock), pump failure or obstruction in the circulatory system (cardiogenic shock), severe allergic reaction (anaphylactic shock), or disruption of the nervous system (neurogenic shock).

Risk factors

- Inter-current heart disease (cardiogenic shock)
- Thromboembolism and amniotic fluid embolism (cardiogenic shock)
- Non-obstetric infections and genital tract sepsis (septic shock)
- Trauma (hypovolaemic shock)

- Obstetric haemorrhage (hypovolaemic shock)
- Inverted uterus (neurogenic or hypovolaemic shock)
- Ruptured ectopic pregnancy (hypovolaemic shock)
- Incomplete miscarriage (neurogenic or hypovolaemic shock)
- Opiate-induced histamine release or other drug allergy (anaphylactic shock)

> **TOP TIP**
>
> **The normal physiological changes of pregnancy (increased plasma and red cell volume) allow the patient to compensate for some time. This can make diagnosis difficult as changes in vital signs may be minimal. Always have a high index of suspicion for concealed internal haemorrhage.**

Diagnosis

In PPH and trauma to the genital tract, external haemorrhage will be obvious and the volume of blood seen may give an indication of the amount of blood lost. However, even in PPH some of the bleeding may be concealed.

In ruptured ectopic pregnancy and placental abruption, almost all of the blood lost may be internal and concealed. As obstetric patients will initially compensate for hypovolaemia, the pre-hospital practitioner must obtain a good history that may, if abnormal, raise the suspicion that concealed haemorrhage may be present.

See Table 7.1 for a summary of the differential diagnosis of shock in the obstetric patient.

> **TOP TIP**
>
> **The main mechanism of maintaining maternal circulation in the event of blood loss is the restriction of blood flow to the uterus. This can occur rapidly following the onset of significant bleeding, and will result in a reduction in placental perfusion with associated fetal hypoxia. Consequently, even in the absence of signs of shock, control of haemorrhage and restoration of circulating volume have the highest priority.**

Table 7.1 Differential diagnosis of shock in the obstetric patient

Aetiology	Pulse rate	BP	Gestation	Blood loss	Other key features
Ruptured ectopic	↑	↓	First trimester (but may not know they are pregnant)	+++ (but probably concealed)	Peritonism; consider possibility in **any** woman of childbearing years with unexplained shock and abdominal pain
Cervical shock	↓	↓	Usually first trimester	+	History suggestive of miscarriage
Antepartum haemorrhage	↑	↓	Second and third trimester	+++ (but may be concealed)	Known placenta praevia; trauma to abdomen, possibly woody uterus
Uterine rupture	↑ or ↓	↓	Labour	+++ (but may be concealed)	History of uterine surgery (caesarean section, fibroids); abdominal trauma
Amniotic fluid embolism/ pulmonary embolism	↑	↓	Advanced or rapid labour	None	Suspect in any patient in advanced labour with sudden collapse including hypoxia and cardiovascular compromise in the absence of any other likely diagnosis
Uterine inversion	↓	↓	Third stage of labour	+	Visible uterus at introitus; may have resulted from cord traction ('managed third stage')
Postpartum haemorrhage (PPH)	↑	↓	Postpartum	+ to +++	Primary PPH associated with perineal and vaginal trauma; secondary PPH may be associated with sepsis; either may be associated with retained placenta/parts
Anaphylaxis	↑	↓	Any	None	Allergen related (history of atopy); may be drug related – think morphine/opiates

Pre-hospital management

General principles

1. Remember to apply manual uterine displacement or position the mother in the 15–30° left lateral position to avoid further compromise of the fetal circulation due to aortocaval compression by the uterus.
2. Open, clear and secure the airway in accordance with the patient's clinical need.
3. If oxygen saturation on air falls below 94% give oxygen. If SpO_2 is less than 85% use a non-rebreathing mask; otherwise use a simple face mask. Aim for a target saturation of 94–98%.
4. Start transportation without delay to a hospital with obstetric theatres, blood transfusion, intensive care unit (ICU) and anaesthetic services immediately available.
5. Inform the senior on-call obstetrician of your impending arrival.
6. Insert two of the largest bore cannulae possible en route (do NOT delay on scene to do this). Access above the level of the diaphragm is recommended. If it is not possible to gain intravenous access, consider using the intraosseous route.
7. In hypovolaemia, septic shock, neurogenic shock and anaphylaxis only: administer crystalloids in 250 ml aliquots to maintain a systolic BP of 90 mmHg. Apply caution with administering fluids if the systolic BP is 90 mmHg or above to reduce the risk of rebleeding due to clot disruption unless there is other evidence of significant haemorrhage, such as:
   - More than 500 ml of external haemorrhage
   - Altered mental status
   - Dysrhythmias
8. Administer analgesia if the patient is in pain – use morphine cautiously if the patient is hypotensive; consider using paracetamol IV (see Figure 7.4 for the shock algorithm).

TOP TIP

In the pre-hospital setting excessive intravenous fluids should be avoided in cases of cardiogenic shock as administration can cause fluid overload and worsen pulmonary oedema.

Specific management

Hypovolaemic shock

'You cannot treat what you cannot see' is a very basic maxim that requires the practitioner to search for a focus of blood loss. Proper examination of the uterus and external genitalia must be considered in all shocked patients where hypovolaemia is believed to be the cause.

Whilst fluid replacement buys time in the pre-hospital environment, the use of non-blood products facilitates a physiological anaemia. Early blood administration is a key element in the successful resuscitation of the hypovolaemic patient (Battaloglu and Porter, 2016).

The early administration of Tranexamic Acid (within 3 hours of delivery) has been shown to reduce mortality from PPH, following the initial administration of a uterotonic agent. The dosage of Tranexamic Acid is 1g IV, followed by a further dose if bleeding continues, or restarts after 30 minutes (Roberts et al., 2011).

We consider it advisable to administer Tranexamic Acid, where indicated, to both pregnant and post-natal women.

Local guidelines will determine the route and dosage.

A pelvic binder device should be considered in all pregnant trauma patients, and should be applied during the primary survey, when assessing and rectifying 'circulation'.

Cardiogenic shock

Provide supportive treatment in response to clinical signs. Treat dysrhythmias according to usual Resuscitation Council (UK) guidelines.

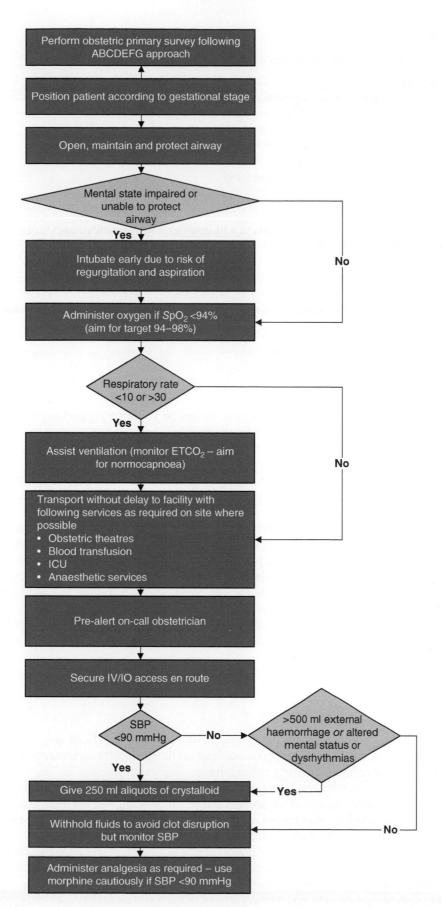

Figure 7.4 Shock algorithm

Anaphylactic shock

Treat in accordance with normal pre-hospital guidelines:

1. Establish a patent airway.
2. Give high-flow oxygen via a non-rebreathing mask.
3. Give adrenaline (1:1000) 500 micrograms IM (repeated after 5 minutes if no improvement).
4. IV fluid challenge 500–1000 ml to maintain the blood pressure.
5. Administer hydrocortisone 200 mg IM or slow IV injection after the initial resuscitation.
6. Give chlorphenamine 10 mg IM or slow IV injection after the initial resuscitation.
7. The use of a salbutamol 5 mg nebuliser can be considered.

TOP TIP

Spending time on scene to cannulate and give fluids to a haemorrhaging obstetric patient is not the best use of time and reduces the probability of survival for the mother and fetus.

TOP TIP

The most effective treatment of obstetric haemorrhage is surgery in an appropriately equipped and staffed maternity theatre suite.

Summary of key points

In cardiac arrest:

- Resuscitation following maternal cardiac arrest should always be commenced and never terminated in the pre-hospital setting, even if the probability of survival for the mother is minimal, to maximise the chances of survival for both the mother and fetus
- Cardiac arrest victims beyond 20 weeks of pregnancy must NOT be managed in the supine position. The uterus should be displaced manually or instead they should be secured to a spine board tilted 15–30° to the patient's left
- Tracheal intubation, using Sellick's manoeuvre, should be performed as quickly as possible to minimise the risk of aspiration
- Ventilation of the obtunded pregnant patient must always be via a cuffed airway device when possible
- Ventilation to compression ratios, defibrillation electrode placement and energy settings, and drug doses are the same for obstetric patients as non-obstetric patients
- The most common presenting cardiac arrest rhythm in pregnancy is pulseless electrical activity
- The decision to move the patient must be taken early in the resuscitation attempt to permit emergency RH/PMCS and to maximise the probability of maternal and fetal survival
- CPR should be continued throughout transfer to hospital where the decision to proceed to RH/PMCS will be made
- Spending time on scene to cannulate and give fluids to a haemorrhaging obstetric patient wastes time and reduces the probability of survival of the mother and fetus
- When informing the hospital about the transfer, remember to recommend that an obstetrician should be in attendance when you arrive at the hospital

In shock:

- The normal physiological changes of pregnancy (increased plasma and red cell volume) allow the patient to compensate for some time. This can make diagnosis difficult as changes in vital signs may be minimal. Always have a high index of suspicion for concealed internal haemorrhage
- The main mechanism of maintaining maternal circulation in the event of blood loss is the restriction of blood flow to the uterus. This can occur rapidly following the onset of significant bleeding, and will result in a reduction in placental perfusion with associated fetal hypoxia. Consequently, even in the absence of signs of shock, control of haemorrhage and restoration of circulating volume have the highest priority
- In the haemorrhaging obstetric patient use 250 ml aliquots of crystalloid to maintain a systolic blood pressure of 90 mmHg
- In the pre-hospital setting, intravenous fluids should be avoided in cases of cardiogenic shock as administration can cause fluid overload and worsen pulmonary oedema
- Opioids, including morphine, cause histamine release; in a small proportion of patients this can lead to anaphylactic reactions
- The most effective treatment of obstetric haemorrhage is usually surgery in an appropriately equipped and staffed maternity theatre suite

CHAPTER 8
Emergencies in early pregnancy (up to 20 weeks)

Learning outcomes

After reading this chapter, you will be able to:
- Describe the pre-hospital management of miscarriage and cervical shock and ectopic pregnancy

Any vaginal bleeding during early pregnancy is abnormal and is a concern to the woman and her partner, especially if there is a history of pregnancy loss; 15–20% of pregnancies result in miscarriage and can cause considerable distress (NICE, 2014). Reassurance and empathy are important elements of caring for the woman; sensitivity to the situation is paramount. There are many causes of vaginal bleeding in early pregnancy, some of which may occasionally lead to life-threatening situations (Marshall and Rayner, 2014). Early pregnancy loss accounts for 50 000 hospital admissions annually in the UK (NICE, 2012).

8.1 Miscarriage

Definition

Miscarriage is the loss of a pregnancy before 24 completed weeks. It can occur in either the first or second trimester. Miscarriage is more common in the first 12 weeks. The further advanced the pregnancy, the more bleeding can occur.

There are different types of spontaneous miscarriage, all of which are associated with vaginal bleeding but may or may not have abdominal pain:

- *Inevitable:* the cervix opens and all products of conception are passed. Bleeding can be heavy or light. If some of the products of conception remain in the uterus, this is classed as an *incomplete miscarriage* and there is increased risk of infection (Marshall and Raynor, 2014)
- *Complete:* all the placental/fetal tissue has passed and the cervix will be closed or closing and bleeding will be settling
- *Threatened:* there has been some bleeding but no tissue has been passed, the cervix remains closed and on ultrasound assessment the fetus is thought to still be viable. It may or may not be accompanied by abdominal pain (Marshall and Raynor, 2014)
- *Missed:* there has been very little or no bleeding but on ultrasound assessment the fetus is either dead or has not developed properly. Products of conception may not be passed spontaneously. This – and incomplete miscarriage – may be managed medically in hospital with between 600 and 800 micrograms of misoprostol (pessary or oral)

Pre-Obstetric Emergency Training: A Practical Approach, Second Edition. Edited by Mark Woolcock.
© 2019 John Wiley & Sons Ltd. Published 2019 by John Wiley & Sons Ltd.

Risk factors

- Previous history of miscarriage
- Previously identified potential miscarriage at scan
- Smoking
- Obesity
- Drug misuse in pregnancy
- Increasing age (rate of miscarriage is 1:10 in women <30 years and 1:2 for women >45 years)
- Alcohol use (more than 2 units per week) (NHS Choices, 2015a)

Diagnosis

Take a clinical history:

- Bleeding can be light or very heavy
- There may be a history of passing clots or jelly-like tissue. Any tissue that has been passed and collected should be brought to hospital. Pregnancy remains are regarded as tissues of the woman and as such the woman has a right to decide how the remains of pregnancy are disposed of and should be involved in any decisions regarding this (HTA, 2015)
- Pain – central, period-like cramps, can radiate to the back or down the legs
- Symptoms of pregnancy may be subsiding such as nausea or breast tenderness

To make an accurate diagnosis of the type of miscarriage, vaginal examination and ultrasound are required; neither is appropriate in the pre-obstetric setting. In the acute situation, management depends on the clinical situation rather than the absolute diagnosis.

Be aware that infection may follow any miscarriage. It can be associated with incomplete miscarriage, post-surgical evacuation or following termination of pregnancy.

> **TOP TIP**
>
> **Any tissue that has been passed and collected should be brought to hospital.**

Pre-hospital management

If there is light bleeding or bleeding that has resolved, with no associated pain, consideration may be given to arranging an appointment in either an outpatient or early pregnancy assessment unit.

In the event of life-threatening bleeding with evidence of confirmed miscarriage (e.g. a patient has been discharged home following medical management and starts to bleed heavily), an oxytocic drug such as ergometrine or syntometrine can be given. Alternatively, misoprostol 800 micrograms PR can be given. (See Chapter 7 for management of shock.) For heavy or life-threatening bleeding, referral to a hospital emergency department with appropriate surgical facilities is required.

> **TOP TIP**
>
> **If shock is out of proportion to bleeding consider ectopic pregnancy or cervical shock.**

> **TOP TIP**
>
> **Periods can be late on occasion. To determine pregnancy ask:**
>
> - **Is the bleeding like a normal period?**
> - **Was the last menstrual period less than 6 weeks ago?**
> - **Has there been a positive pregnancy test?**

8.2 Cervical shock

This occurs when some products of conception partially pass through the cervix and become 'trapped', causing stimulation of the vagus nerve and subsequent symptomatic bradycardia and hypotension. The level of shock is often out of proportion to the amount of blood loss (JRCALC, 2016).

> **TOP TIP**
>
> **Cervical shock is a life-threatening emergency that requires urgent obstetric intervention to resolve. These patients should be transported to hospital without delay, with IV fluids given en route to maintain systolic BP above 90 mmHg and consideration given to the use of doses of 500 micrograms atropine to manage bradycardia.**

8.3 Ectopic pregnancy

Definition

An ectopic pregnancy occurs when a fertilised ovum implants somewhere other than in the uterine cavity – normally (97% of cases) in the fallopian tube (Fellowes and Woolcock, 2008), but it can rarely implant on the ovary or elsewhere in the abdominal cavity (Figure 8.1). Ectopic pregnancy occurs in 11:1000 pregnancies (Elson et al., 2016), with the mortality being 0.2 in 1000 pregnancies (NICE, 2012). However, morbidity from ectopic pregnancy has reduced in recent years, possibly through improved diagnosis and treatment (Elson et al., 2016). The symptoms initially are often vague and a high index of suspicion is required. NICE state that during clinical assessment of women of reproductive age, be aware that:

- the woman may be pregnant; think about offering a pregnancy test even when symptoms are non-specific **and**
- the symptoms and signs of ectopic pregnancy can resemble the common symptoms and signs of other conditions, for example gastrointestinal conditions or urinary tract infection (NICE, 2012)

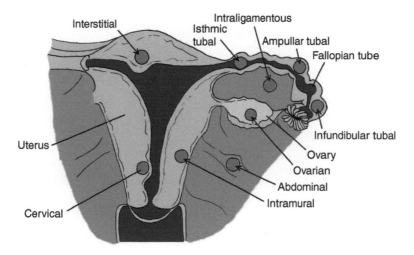

Figure 8.1 Possible sites of ectopic implantation

Risk factors

- Pelvic inflammatory disease (PID) or sexually transmitted infection (particularly *Chlamydia*)
- Previous tubal surgery
- Infertility or women undergoing treatment for infertility
- Smoking
- Use of intrauterine device contraceptive
- Previous ectopic pregnancy
- Sterilisation or reversal of sterilisation
- Endometriosis
- Uterine fibroids

However, one-third of patients do not have any known risk factors (NICE, 2012).

Diagnosis

Clinical history

The patient is usually 6–8 weeks' pregnant, but may not be aware of or may deny pregnancy, and may complain of some of the following:

- Vaginal bleeding with or without clots
- Amenorrhoea or missed period
- Pelvic or abdominal pain
- Breast tenderness
- Gastrointestinal symptoms
- Shoulder tip pain
- Urinary symptoms
- Passage of tissue
- Rectal pressure or pain on defecation

> **TOP TIP**
>
> **Have a high index of suspicion for ectopic pregnancy in any woman of childbearing age with a history of abdominal pain, fainting, collapse or signs of shock out of proportion with the amount of blood loss.**

> **TOP TIP**
>
> **Cardiovascular instability should be taken seriously. Women who die of ectopic pregnancy die from blood loss; urgent action is indicated in such cases.**

Examination findings

- Pelvic/abdominal/adnexal tenderness (tenderness over the ovary/fallopian tubes/broad ligaments) that is often localised unilaterally
- Rebound tenderness
- Abdominal distension
- Vaginal bleeding (this may be absent)
- Pallor
- Tachycardia (>100 bpm)
- Hypotension (<100/60 mmHg)
- Orthostatic hypotension
- Breathlessness/tachypnoea
- Shock or collapse

> **TOP TIP**
>
> **Bleeding associated with ectopic pregnancy:**
>
> - **Is often lighter than a period**
> - **Is often unilateral**
> - **May be associated with shoulder tip pain**
> - **May be associated with diarrhoea**

> **TOP TIP**
>
> **An ectopic pregnancy can present with atypical urinary or bowel symptoms (e.g. diarrhoea, pain on defecation). Maternal deaths from ruptured ectopic pregnancies have occurred when these symptoms were ignored (CMACE, 2011).**

Biochemical markers

There will be women being monitored in the community with serial beta human chorionic gonadotrophin (β-hCG) measurements who are considered to be at risk of ectopic pregnancy. Check with the patient to determine if this is the case.

TOP TIP

Ectopic pregnancy is often asymptomatic up to 4–6 weeks' gestation. Ultrasound scan is the primary method of diagnosis.

The fact that a period has not been missed does not exclude an ectopic pregnancy, but on closer questioning the last period was often lighter than normal.

Pre-hospital management

Depending on the setting in which the patient is encountered, many women can be referred to an early pregnancy assessment service (or out-of-hours service) if they present with abdominal or pelvic pain and tenderness, and have a positive pregnancy test with no other symptoms. If ectopic pregnancy is suspected or the woman is unwell, a referral to a hospital emergency department with access to obstetric and gynaecology services is always appropriate.

TOP TIP

All healthcare professionals involved in the care of women of reproductive age should have access to pregnancy tests (NICE, 2012). In many cases for pre-hospital providers this can only be achieved through referral to hospital for assessment.

8.4 Pre-hospital management of complications in early pregnancy

1. Perform an obstetric primary survey following an ABCDEFG approach; address life-threatening findings in priority order.
2. Consider the patient's position according to gestational stage and presenting condition.
3. Give oxygen if SpO_2 (on air) falls below 94%; aim for a target saturation of 94–98%.
4. Assess and document vital signs: respiratory rate, oxygen saturation, pulse rate (including quality), capillary refill time (CRT) or blood pressure, conscious level, temperature and blood glucose level.
5. Take a detailed obstetric history (if patient's condition allows); request/review hand-held notes where possible.
6. Assess and document quantity of blood loss:
   - Blood at the toes
   - Blood loss on pad
   - Blood on clothes
   - Blood on bed sheets
7. Transport without delay to the appropriate hospital facility if significant blood loss is found or suspected: the emergency department for ectopic/life-threatening miscarriage or cervical shock. For lower acuity problems, manage as per agreed local pathways (emergency department or other outpatient facility such as an early pregnancy assessment unit).
8. Consider pre-alert based on the patient's condition.
9. Obtain IV access (largest possible) en route to hospital if the patient is showing signs of, or in anticipation of, shock (pallor, tachypnoea, hypotension, tachycardia or bradycardia). Consider subtle signs such as the patient reporting feeling cold or thirsty, sweaty or clammy, anxiety or postural hypotension.
10. Commence IV fluid (250 ml aliquots) to maintain a systolic BP of 90 mmHg (JRCALC, 2016).
11. Administer analgesia as appropriate; apply caution when planning to administer morphine to a hypotensive patient. Consider IV paracetamol. Do not forget Entonox® as an effective analgesic.
12. Bradycardia secondary to cervical shock can be treated with IV atropine (500 micrograms repeated up to 3 mg).
13. Life-threatening haemorrhage in the case of **confirmed** miscarriage (where the patient has been discharged home with medical management and starts to bleed) may require an oxytocic drug, as per local clinical guidelines. **If there is any doubt about the possible viability of the fetus, do not administer such a drug.**

Summary of key points

In miscarriage:

- Cervical shock is a life-threatening emergency that requires urgent obstetric intervention to resolve. These patients should be transported to hospital without delay with IV fluids given en route
- Any tissue that has been passed and collected should be brought to the hospital
- If shock is out of proportion to bleeding consider ectopic or cervical shock
- In the event of life-threatening bleeding and miscarriage has been confirmed (or medically managed) an oxytocic drug should be administered
- Alternatively, misoprostol PR can be given

In ectopic pregnancy:

- No single component is likely to diagnose an ectopic pregnancy in isolation – the complete picture is more important
- Have a high index of suspicion for ectopic pregnancy in any woman of childbearing age with history of abdominal pain, fainting, collapse or signs of shock out of proportion with blood loss
- An absence of amenorrhoea does not exclude an ectopic pregnancy but on closer questioning the last period was often lighter than normal
- Ectopic pregnancy can present with atypical urinary or bowel symptoms (e.g. diarrhoea, pain on defecation). Maternal deaths from ruptured ectopic pregnancies have occurred when these symptoms were ignored
- If already shocked, ectopic pregnancy is a life-threatening situation and speed is of the essence; a full history from a family member en route is always useful in these situations. Emergency transfer with an pre-alert call is required
- Vaginal bleeding can be absent, light or heavy in ectopic pregnancy, although heavier loss is more often associated with miscarriage

CHAPTER 9
Emergencies in late pregnancy (from 20 weeks)

Learning outcomes

After reading this chapter, you will be able to define, identify and describe the pre-hospital management of:
- Pregnancy-induced hypertension (PIH), pre-eclampsia and eclampsia, haemolysis, elevated liver enzymes and low platelets (HELLP) syndrome and acute fatty liver of pregnancy (AFLP)
- Antepartum haemorrhage (APH), including placenta praevia and placental abruption
- Uterine rupture
- Amniotic fluid embolus

This chapter addresses the recognition and management of emergencies in the later stages of pregnancy, including the first and second stages of labour – up to and including delivery of the baby.

9.1 Hypertension in pregnancy

Hypertension from all causes is the commonest medical problem in pregnancy and affects between 10% and 15% of all pregnancies. Hypertensive conditions include PIH, pre-existing hypertension (e.g. 'essential' hypertension), pre-eclampsia and eclampsia. The two conditions of HELLP syndrome and AFLP are felt to be part of the spectrum of disease that includes pre-eclampsia and eclampsia.

Pre-existing hypertension

Definition

Women may enter pregnancy with pre-existing hypertension. If hypertension is detected before 20 weeks, this is likely to reflect pre-existing hypertension. Hypertension in a young person may only be detected for the first time in early pregnancy. At some point, this will require formal investigation to exclude an underlying cause (e.g. renal or cardiac disease, or Cushing's syndrome). However, most will not have a defined cause and fall under the category of mild 'essential' hypertension. These women are at increased risk of developing superimposed pre-eclampsia and fetal growth restriction. The risk is almost 50% if there is severe hypertension in early pregnancy (diastolic BP >110 mmHg, systolic BP >160 mmHg). Again, such patients require close monitoring in order to detect complications, and in particular the development of pre-eclampsia or growth restriction.

Pre-Obstetric Emergency Training: A Practical Approach, Second Edition. Edited by Mark Woolcock.
© 2019 John Wiley & Sons Ltd. Published 2019 by John Wiley & Sons Ltd.

Pregnancy-induced hypertension

Definition

Pregnancy-induced hypertension is a significant rise in blood pressure occurring after 20 weeks in the **absence of proteinuria or other features of pre-eclampsia**. Women with uncomplicated PIH require close monitoring in the antenatal period to pick up those who are going to develop pre-eclampsia. If hypertension is uncomplicated by pre-eclampsia, the maternal and fetal outcomes are good.

Pre-eclampsia

Definition

Pre-eclampsia is hypertension associated with proteinuria developing after 20 weeks' gestation. It can occur as early as 20 weeks but more commonly occurs in the third trimester. It is more common in first pregnancies where one in ten women will develop pre-eclampsia. **Severe pre-eclampsia** is pre-eclampsia with severe hypertension (>160/110 mmHg) and/or with symptoms and/or haematological impairment. The incidence of severe pre-eclampsia is approximately 1% of all pregnancies.

The underlying pathophysiology is not fully understood. However, it is known that the placenta plays an important role, such that the normal physiological changes that occur in the vessels of the uterus do not occur. This leads to poor perfusion of the placenta, resulting in a fetus which is growth restricted.

In the 2013–15 report, pre-eclampsia accounted for 3 of the 88 maternal deaths related to direct pregnancy causes (MBRRACE-UK, 2017). In previous reports, the care of 70% of women who died was deemed to be substandard, and these deaths may have been avoided with better care (CMACE, 2011).

Risk factors for pre-eclampsia and eclampsia

- Primigravidity or first child with a new partner
- Previous severe pre-eclampsia
- Essential hypertension
- Diabetes
- Obesity
- Twins or higher multiples
- Renal disease
- Advanced maternal age (over 40 years)
- Young maternal age (less than 16 years)
- Pre-existing cardiovascular disease
- Cushing's disease

Diagnosis

Women with mild to moderate pre-eclampsia are asymptomatic and the disease is usually diagnosed at routine antenatal visits. This is often managed on an outpatient basis initially, with regular review on the obstetric day unit. However, it may require admission to hospital and early delivery if the disease progresses.

TOP TIP

In the UK, the diagnosis of pre-eclampsia includes an increase in blood pressure (above 140/90 mmHg) and detection of protein in the urine.

When measuring BP, the woman should be semi-recumbent and an appropriately sized cuff should be used. In women with a larger arm, using a normal-sized cuff may result in falsely high BP readings. It is important to record both systolic and diastolic pressures. The latter should be assessed using Korotkoff V (that is, sound disappearance). Korotkoff IV (that is, 'muffling') should only be used if heart sounds do not disappear as pressure readings fall to zero (see Chapter 5).

Severe pre-eclampsia may present in a patient with known mild pre-eclampsia or may present with little prior warning. The BP is significantly raised (<160/110 mmHg) with proteinuria and/or more of the following symptoms and signs:

- Headache – severe and frontal
- Visual disturbances (such as blurring or flashing)
- Papilloedema
- Epigastric pain (due to stretching of the liver capsule) – often mistaken for heartburn
- Right-sided upper abdominal pain – due to stretching of the liver capsule
- Muscle twitching or tremor
- Other symptoms – nausea, vomiting, confusion
- Rapidly progressive oedema

Severe pre-eclampsia is a 'multi-organ' disease – although hypertension is a cardinal feature, other complications include:

- Intracranial haemorrhage
- Stroke
- Renal failure
- Liver failure
- Abnormal blood clotting such as disseminated intravascular coagulation (DIC)
- Placental abruption and associated massive haemorrhage

One of the 'top ten recommendations' in the CEMACH report highlighted the importance of aggressive treatment of high systolic BP (160 mmHg or more) in order to reduce the chance of maternal intracerebral bleeding and stroke (CEMACH, 2007b). Therefore, these obstetric patients require immediate admission to an appropriate obstetric unit.

Pre-hospital management

Pre-hospital healthcare practitioners will not usually be involved with management of gestational hypertension or mild pre-eclampsia. However, it is important that any pregnant woman should have their BP checked during assessment, even if they do not have suspicious symptoms. A new finding of a BP of 140/90 or higher requires review by a midwife or discussion with the local obstetric unit to decide if admission is necessary.

> **TOP TIP**
>
> **A new systolic BP of 150 or a diastolic BP of 100 or higher should trigger admission to an obstetric unit.**

The following recommendations relate to the management of women with severe pre-eclampsia:

1. Perform an obstetric primary survey following an ABCDEFG approach; address life-threatening findings in priority order.
2. Consider the patient's position according to gestational stage and presenting condition.
3. Give oxygen if SpO_2 (on air) falls below 94%; aim for a target saturation of 94–98%.
4. Assess for any 'time-critical' features requiring immediate transfer:
   - Headache – severe and frontal
   - Visual disturbances
   - Epigastric pain
   - Right-sided upper abdominal pain
   - Muscle twitching or tremor
   - Confusion
5. Secure venous access en route to the hospital in case IV medication is required (see Eclampsia section).
6. **DO NOT** give routine IV fluids as these patients are at risk of developing acute pulmonary oedema, even with small boluses of crystalloid. If fluids are attached to the cannula, the flow rate should be no more than 80 ml/h (use normal saline or Hartmann's, but not dextrose in water).
7. **Measure blood pressure continually** (the aim is for a BP of 150/80–100 mmHg).
8. Provide the receiving hospital with a pre-alert message.
9. Assess and document all other vital signs: respiratory rate, oxygen saturation, pulse rate (including quality), conscious level, temperature and blood glucose level.
10. Take a detailed obstetric history (if patient's condition allows); request hand-held notes where possible as a review of these will highlight any changes in BP over the preceding weeks.

> **TOP TIP**
>
> **Do not give IV fluids until necessary. Restrict IV fluids to a maximum of 80 ml/h to avoid pulmonary oedema.**
>
> **Avoid ergometrine/syntometrine in the third stage of labour, as it may precipitate severe hypertension and intracerebral bleeding.**

Eclampsia

Definition

Eclampsia is defined as tonic-clonic, generalised 'grand mal' seizures, usually in association with signs or symptoms of pre-eclampsia. It is one of the most dangerous complications of pregnancy, with a mortality rate of 2% in the UK. It occurs in 2.7:10 000 deliveries, usually beyond 24 weeks (Knight, 2007). Many patients will have had pre-existing pre-eclampsia (of mild, moderate or severe degree), **but cases of eclampsia can present acutely with no prior warning**. One-third of cases present for the first time post-delivery (usually in the first 48 hours).

Although eclampsia is often preceded by severe pre-eclampsia, in many cases the blood pressure will only be mildly elevated at presentation.

The hypoxia caused during a grand mal seizure may lead to significant fetal compromise and even death. There is a risk of placental abruption and massive haemorrhage. Occasionally, there may be cortical blindness after an eclamptic fit. Fitting is usually self-limiting, but may be prolonged and repeated.

Other complications associated with eclampsia include renal failure, hepatic failure and DIC.

> **TOP TIP**
>
> **Always assume that a tonic-clonic seizure in pregnancy (beyond 20 weeks) is due to eclampsia until proven otherwise.**

Diagnosis

The diagnosis is made through the presence or history of a tonic-clonic fit after 20 weeks of pregnancy.

> **TOP TIP**
>
> **Epileptic patients can have tonic-clonic fits. If after 20 weeks of pregnancy a fitting epileptic patient has a history of hypertension or pre-eclampsia, treat as for eclampsia. If there is no hypertension or pre-eclampsia, treat for epilepsy, but monitor the blood pressure until after the postictal phase and discuss with the midwife.**

Pre-hospital management

1. Perform an obstetric primary survey following an ABCDEFG approach; address life-threatening findings in priority order.
2. Consider the patient's position according to gestational stage and presenting condition.
3. Give oxygen if SpO_2 (on air) falls below 94%; aim for a target saturation of 94–98%.
4. If the mother has continuous or recurrent fits at scene, secure IV or IO access. Otherwise postpone obtaining access until en route to the hospital.
5. This is a time-critical situation and transport to the hospital should be arranged at the earliest opportunity.
6. Provide the receiving hospital with a pre-alert message.
7. **If magnesium sulphate is unavailable and the patient is in status epilepticus**, consider Diazemuls® 10–20 mg IV or IO, or rectal diazepam 10–20 mg, titrated against effect.
8. The definitive treatment of eclampsia, either to treat ongoing or recurrent fits, or to prevent further fits occurring, is magnesium sulphate 4 g loading dose IV or IO over 10 minutes (this would then be followed by an infusion of 1 g/h for 24 hours in hospital).
9. Assess and document vital signs: respiratory rate, oxygen saturation, pulse rate (including quality), CRT or blood pressure, conscious level, temperature and blood glucose level.
10. Take a detailed obstetric history (if patient's condition allows); request/review hand-held notes where possible.

TOP TIP

Usually, eclamptic fits are single and self-limiting, lasting for approximately 2 minutes. The definitive treatment is magnesium sulphate to prevent further fits.

If magnesium sulphate is unavailable, avoid using diazepam or other benzodiazepines unless the fit reoccurs (Figure 9.1).

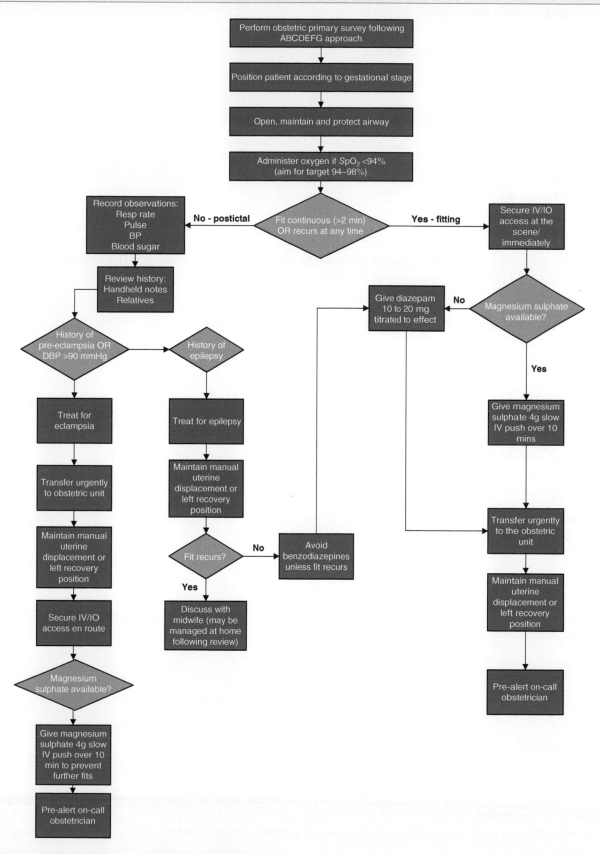

Figure 9.1 Management of convulsions in pregnancy

HELLP syndrome

Definition

This is a syndrome related to pre-eclampsia (haemolysis, elevated liver enzymes and low platelets). It is more common in multigravid patients, and presents with:

- Hypertension
- Right upper quadrant or epigastric pain (65%)
- Nausea and vomiting (35%)
- Placental abruption (15%)
- Liver rupture (rare)

Risk factors

- Known pre-eclampsia
- Multiparity
- Previous history of HELLP

Diagnosis

This will not be diagnosed in the pre-hospital setting; however, you may have a suspicion based on symptoms.

Pre-hospital management

Management in the pre-hospital situation is the same as for severe pre-eclampsia.

Acute fatty liver of pregnancy

Definition

Acute fatty liver of pregnancy is a rare condition (1:10 000 pregnancies) but has a high maternal mortality (10–20%) and fetal mortality (20–30%). Presentation is usually nearer 37 weeks and the cardinal symptom is severe nausea, vomiting, malaise and mild jaundice. Features of mild pre-eclampsia may be present. Pre-hospital care is the same as for severe pre-eclampsia. Management in hospital is supportive with prompt delivery (induction of labour or caesarean section).

Risk factors

- First pregnancy
- Obesity
- Male fetus

Diagnosis

This will not be diagnosed in the pre-hospital setting; however, you may have a suspicion based on symptoms. A low blood glucose level would raise the index of suspicion.

Pre-hospital management

Management in the pre-hospital situation is the same as for severe pre-eclampsia.

9.2 Antepartum haemorrhage

Definition

Antepartum haemorrhage is defined as bleeding from the vagina before labour but after 24 completed weeks of pregnancy. APH is reported to complicate around 3–5% of all pregnancies (Gorman and Penna, 2015). The volume of blood lost can be just a few millilitres, and in most cases this is not indicative of a serious problem. However, it is vital that even if blood loss is minimal, the patient is assessed and monitored carefully as, occasionally, a small amount of external blood loss may be associated with significant internal (concealed) haemorrhage as in the case of a placental abruption (see Section 9.3).

Significant external haemorrhage of 1 litre or more can also occur, and this is commonly associated with placenta praevia (see Section 9.4). Massive APH is the cause of 13% of stillbirths in the UK (CMACE, 2011) and it still remains an uncommon cause of death in the UK (MBRRACE-UK, 2017). Maternal death from APH is rare – in the period 2008–10, there were only four cases (CMACE, 2011). However, APH can weaken the mother's ability to cope with PPH.

> **TOP TIP**
>
> **A small amount of blood lost externally may indicate a massive concealed haemorrhage: any volume of external blood loss greater than that of a 'show' (i.e. blood loss more than the size of a drink coaster) should alert the practitioner to the risk of serious hidden bleeding.**

Risk factors

- Maternal age over 40 years
- Presence of complex medical disorders before pregnancy
- Multigravida
- Previous caesarean section resulting in placenta praevia or placenta accreta (abnormal adherence of part or all of the placenta to the uterine wall)
- Known placenta praevia
- Previous history of abruption
- Use of crack cocaine, which can precipitate abruption
- Coagulopathies

Diagnosis

External blood loss that even slightly exceeds the quantity of a normal 'show' should be treated with suspicion. A thorough ABCDEFG approach should be applied to patient assessment and ongoing monitoring. The practitioner should anticipate the possibility of a minor bleed being associated with ongoing concealed bleeding or a subsequent catastrophic revealed haemorrhage. If the vital signs indicate shock then this should precipitate appropriate management regardless of the quantity of blood that has been seen; however, up to 35% of the maternal blood volume can be lost without a concomitant fall in blood pressure or increase in heart rate.

> **TOP TIP**
>
> **Obstetric patients may lose up to 35% of their blood volume without a change in their blood pressure or heart rate.**

Pre-hospital management

The generic treatment for APH is the same regardless of whether it is concealed or revealed. **This is a time-critical, life-threatening emergency requiring transport to hospital without unnecessary delay.**

1. Perform an obstetric primary survey following an ABCDEFG approach; address life-threatening findings in priority order.
2. Consider the patient's position according to gestational stage and presenting condition.
3. Give oxygen if SpO_2 (on air) falls below 94%; aim for a target saturation of 94–98%.
4. Transport without delay to a hospital with staffed obstetric theatres, blood transfusion, ICU and anaesthetic services.
5. Provide the receiving hospital with a pre-alert message, ensuring that a senior on-call obstetrician is aware of your impending arrival.
6. Assess and document quantity of blood loss:
   - Blood at the toes
   - Blood loss on pad
   - Blood on clothes
   - Blood on bed sheets
7. Insert one or two large-bore cannulae en route (do NOT delay on scene to do this). If it is not possible to gain IV access, consider using the IO route.

8. Administer crystalloids in 250 ml aliquots to maintain a systolic BP of >90 mmHg. Do NOT administer further 250 ml aliquots once the systolic BP reaches >90 mmHg as this may increase the risk of rebleeding due to clot disruption. Watch closely for further signs of circulatory decompensation.
9. Assess and document vital signs: respiratory rate, oxygen saturation, pulse rate (including quality), CRT or blood pressure, conscious level, temperature and blood glucose level.
10. Administer analgesia as appropriate; apply caution when planning to administer morphine to a hypotensive patient.
11. Take a detailed obstetric history (if patient's condition allows); request/review hand-held notes where possible.

> **TOP TIP**
>
> **Do NOT delay on scene trying to secure IV access: the treatment of massive APH is surgery.**

> **TOP TIP**
>
> **Hypotensive resuscitation is NOT appropriate in managing hypovolaemic shock in obstetric patients.**

> **TOP TIP**
>
> **The three interventions most likely to save the lives of the mother and baby are:**
>
> 1. **Immediate transportation**
> 2. **Selecting a receiving hospital with staffed obstetric theatres, blood transfusion, ICU and anaesthetic services immediately available**
> 3. **Pre-alerting the senior on-call obstetrician**

> **TOP TIP**
>
> **Have a high index of suspicion of concealed haemorrhage in the presence of an appropriate history and altered mental status or dysrhythmias (particularly worsening tachycardia) regardless of the systolic BP.**

9.3 Placental abruption

Definition

Placental abruption is defined as separation of a normally sited placenta from the uterine wall, resulting in bleeding from the maternal sinuses. Haemorrhage is commonly entirely or partially concealed, as blood can only escape through the genital canal if it tracks down behind the membranes. The muscle wall of the uterus itself can also be infiltrated with blood (Couvelaire uterus). However, total blood loss is likely to be significant. The severity of shock can be sufficiently severe to result in maternal coagulopathies (e.g. DIC) and renal failure. Three women died of abruption between 2013 and 2015 (MBRRACE-UK, 2017).

Risk factors

- Maternal age over 40 years
- Presence of complex medical disorders before pregnancy
- Multigravida
- Previous history of abruption
- Use of crack cocaine, which can precipitate abruption
- Coagulopathies
- Gestational hypertension or pre-eclampsia
- Road traffic collisions/significant abdominal trauma

Diagnosis

Conduct a thorough ABCDEFG primary survey and obtain an obstetric history: abruption can be associated with hypertension. Note that placental abruption can occur at any point in a pregnancy. In contrast to placenta praevia, an abruption commonly results in very severe abdominal pain. The patient may describe this as a contraction that never goes away. If the patient is not already in labour, contractions are likely to start, but this will be difficult to assess as the uterus is tense and abdominal tenderness will be present. **On palpation the uterus may feel hard and woody**.

The volume of blood lost is likely to be dramatically underestimated; any revealed bleeding may be dark in colour as it may have desaturated during its slowed passage to the cervical canal. The volume of blood lost and the loss of the maternal–fetal circulation arising from significant separation of the placenta can result in intrauterine death (Figure 9.2).

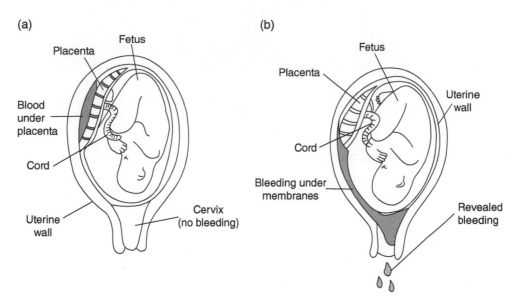

Figure 9.2 (a) Concealed abruption: here all of the bleeding is under the placenta, pain is significant and the uterus tender, with no revealed bleeding. (b) Placental abruption where bleeding is most revealed

> **TOP TIP**
>
> **If the patient appears to be shocked with minimal external haemorrhage and a painful tense ('woody') uterus, always assume placental abruption.**

Pre-hospital management

If you suspect placental abruption, **this is a time-critical emergency: immediate transportation to hospital is vital**. Both mother and baby are at risk, although the baby is likely to die before the mother. Tactfully ask the mother when she last felt the baby move and remember to pass this information to the receiving obstetrician. Follow the generic treatment guidelines for APH (see Section 9.2) and apply a robust ABCDEFG approach.

9.4 Placenta praevia

Definition

Placenta praevia is defined as a placenta completely or partially situated in the lower part of the uterus. Separation of the placenta can occur in late pregnancy due to contractions or sexual intercourse: this causes tearing of blood vessels close to the cervical canal, commonly resulting in vaginal bleeding. Nine deaths from APH resulting from placenta praevia occurred between 2013 and 2015, although of these, five were post caesarean delivery (MBRRACE-UK, 2017) (Figure 9.3).

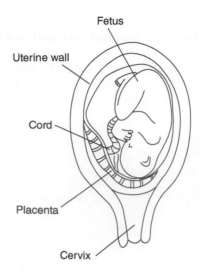

Figure 9.3 Major placenta praevia: low lying placenta

Diagnosis

The volume of revealed blood loss may be significant, particularly if the patient is in labour as this may cause further separation and tearing of blood vessels. The lost blood tends to be bright red. The uterus is relaxed and the abdomen is not tender – indeed the patient may well be pain free if they are not in labour. It should be noted, however, that the bleeding often causes uterine irritation resulting in contractions and therefore pain. Death of the fetus in utero is rare, although malpresentations are common because the low placenta prevents the head engaging in the pelvis.

As always, a thorough ABCDEFG assessment is essential. Obtaining an obstetric history is equally important: placenta praevia is usually identified during routine scans and patients at risk will be booked for an elective caesarean section 14 days before their due delivery date. Recurrent episodic bleeding is common, and the patient may have already been admitted for an APH during the current pregnancy.

Pre-hospital management

If the volume of blood loss is significant or the patient is in shock, **this is a time-critical emergency: immediate transportation to hospital is vital**. Follow the generic treatment guidelines for APH (see Section 9.2).

9.5 Uterine rupture

Definition

Uterine rupture is a tear in the uterus usually associated with previous caesarean section or other uterine surgery such as myomectomy (removal of fibroids). This is rare (incidence of 3:10 000 deliveries) and is most likely to occur during labour. It is a life-threatening emergency for mother and child. Women who have had a previous classic caesarean section (vertical incision of the uterus) are at high risk of uterine rupture and would normally be delivered by planned caesarean section in future pregnancies.

Uterine rupture can also rarely occur after blunt abdominal trauma such as a road traffic collision or domestic violence. Maternal mortality is in the region of 10%, and fetal mortality will approach 100% unless urgent delivery is achieved.

Diagnosis

Uterine rupture may present with:

- Sudden cessation of contractions if in labour
- Elevation (retraction) of the presenting part if in labour
- Vaginal bleeding if in labour
- Severe constant pain
- Fetal distress or death
- Maternal shock due to concealed massive haemorrhage

Pre-hospital management

This is a time-critical, life-threatening emergency requiring immediate transfer to hospital.

Follow the generic treatment for an APH, with maternal resuscitation and immediate transfer to an obstetric unit.

9.6 Amniotic fluid embolus

Definition

An amniotic fluid embolus is defined as the entry into the maternal circulation of amniotic fluid, usually via the placenta. This usually happens towards the end of labour or within 30 minutes of delivery. The amniotic fluid entering the maternal circulation causes cardiovascular collapse and coagulopathy. Although amniotic fluid embolism is rare (the frequency lying between 1.25 and 12.5 per 100 000 maternities), the most recent UK data give an incidence of two per 100 000 (RCOG, 2011). In the 2013–15 reporting period, nine women died from amniotic fluid embolism (MBRRACE-UK, 2017).

Diagnosis

Diagnosis is clinical, and classically presents with an acute fetal distress or maternal collapse characterised by circulatory problems and profound hypoxia, often with seizures or loss of consciousness, and then development of coagulation failure. Major haemorrhage after delivery is common due to coagulopathy. Occasionally, there may be premonitory symptoms up to half an hour before collapse such as feelings of doom, restlessness, altered mental status and breathlessness.

Pre-hospital management

This is a time-critical, life-threatening emergency requiring immediate transfer to hospital.

The patient will require immediate transfer to an obstetric unit. Please refer to the algorithm for managing shock in pregnancy (see Chapter 7, Figure 7.4).

TOP TIP

Suspect amniotic fluid embolus in any patient in advanced labour with sudden collapse, including hypoxia and cardio-vascular compromise, in the absence of any other likely diagnosis.

9.7 Pre-hospital management of shock in late pregnancy

This is a time-critical, life-threatening emergency requiring immediate transfer to hospital.

1. Perform an obstetric primary survey; address life-threatening findings in priority order. Consider early intubation in an obtunded patient due to the high risk of regurgitation and aspiration.
2. Consider the patient's position according to gestational stage and presenting condition.
3. Give oxygen if SpO_2 (on air) falls below 94%; aim for a target saturation of 94–98%.
4. Transport without delay to a hospital with staffed obstetric theatres, blood transfusion, ICU and anaesthetic services.
5. Provide the receiving hospital with a pre-alert message, ensuring that a senior on-call obstetrician is aware of your impending arrival.
6. Insert one or two large-bore cannulae en route (do not delay on scene to do this). If it is not possible to gain IV access, consider using the IO route.

7. Administer crystalloids in 250 ml aliquots to maintain a systolic BP of 90 mmHg. Apply caution when administering fluids if the systolic BP is 90 mmHg to reduce the risk of rebleeding due to clot disruption unless there is evidence of significant haemorrhage, such as:
   • More than 500 ml external haemorrhage, *or*
   • Altered mental status, *or*
   • Dysrhythmias
8. Assess and document vital signs: respiratory rate, oxygen saturation, pulse rate (including quality), CRT or blood pressure, conscious level, temperature and blood glucose level.
9. Administer analgesia as appropriate; apply caution when planning to administer morphine to a hypotensive patient; consider IV paracetamol.
10. Take a detailed obstetric history (if patient's condition allows); request/review hand-held notes where possible.

Summary of key points

In pre-eclampsia and related conditions:

- In the initial stages of pre-eclampsia, women are asymptomatic
- Severe pre-eclampsia is often associated with headaches, visual disturbances and upper abdominal pain (right-sided)
- IV fluids must be restricted in women with pre-eclampsia because of the risk of pulmonary oedema
- Eclamptic fits should be managed like any tonic-clonic seizure, taking particular care to protect the airway by placing the patient in the recovery position (preferably on their left side)
- One-third of cases of eclampsia occur in the postnatal period. This is usually within 6–12 hours of delivery, but there are rare cases in the literature of eclampsia occurring several days post-delivery. This should always be on your differential list of diagnoses if called to see a woman in the community who has suggestive symptoms
- Avoid administering any compound containing ergometrine as this may cause a dangerously high rise in blood pressure

In APH, placenta praevia and placental abruption:

- In APH, a small amount of blood lost externally can still be associated with a large concealed haemorrhage (abruption)
- Up to 35% of the maternal blood volume can be lost without a concomitant fall in blood pressure or increase in heart rate
- Regardless of the nature of the obstetric emergency do NOT be distracted into forgetting to position a patient with a gravid uterus in the 15–30° left lateral position, or utilise manual uterine displacement
- If a patient appears to be shocked with minimal external haemorrhage and a painful tense uterus, always assume placental abruption

In amniotic fluid embolus:

- Suspect amniotic fluid embolus in any patient in advanced labour with sudden collapse, including hypoxia and cardiovascular compromise, in the absence of any other likely diagnosis

CHAPTER 10
Trauma, surgical and medical emergencies

Learning outcomes

After reading this chapter, you will be able to define, identify and describe the pre-hospital management of:
- Cardiac disease in pregnancy
- Epilepsy in pregnancy
- Venous thromboembolism in pregnancy
- Diabetes in pregnancy
- Respiratory disease in pregnancy
- Trauma in pregnancy
- Substance misuse in pregnancy
- Carbon monoxide poisoning in pregnancy
- Rape and sexual assault in pregnancy
- Perinatal psychiatric illness

10.1 Cardiac disease in pregnancy

Definition

Cardiac disease is generally described as congenital or acquired. There are significant physiological changes to the cardiovascular system in pregnancy (see Chapter 5) and obstetric patients with pre-existing cardiac disease may suffer an exacerbation of symptoms as a result. In the period from 2011 to 2013, approximately 23% of all maternal deaths in the UK (49 in total) resulted from cardiac disease (MBRRACE-UK, 2015a), making this the leading indirect cause of death. The majority of these deaths were related to acquired cardiac diseases, the most common of which were classified as sudden adult death syndrome (SADS) (25%), aortic dissection (20%) and peripartum cardiomyopathy (12%); 22% died from other cardiac conditions. Acute coronary syndromes accounted for 20% of all cardiac-related deaths. The 2013–15 MBRRACE-UK report showed a similar trend, noting that cardiac disease remains the leading cause of indirect maternal death during or up to 6 weeks after the end of pregnancy with a rate of 2.34 per 100 000 maternities.

Risk factors

- Pre-existing cardiac disease
- Obesity
- Smoking
- Family history

Pre-Obstetric Emergency Training: A Practical Approach, Second Edition. Edited by Mark Woolcock.
© 2019 John Wiley & Sons Ltd. Published 2019 by John Wiley & Sons Ltd.

- Diabetes
- Hypertension
- Hypercholesterolaemia
- Maternal age over 35 years
- Marfan's syndrome
- Rheumatic fever – a particular risk in patients originating from areas with a higher prevalence

Diagnosis

The symptoms of an acute coronary syndrome (ACS) are the same during pregnancy as they are for any other patient, although distinguishing an acute cardiac cause for chest pain from symptoms related to gastro-oesophageal reflux (common in pregnancy) can be difficult. It should be noted that in normal pregnancy there may be some increased dyspnoea, but radiating, crushing pain is always a 'red flag'. The practitioner must have a high index of suspicion and perform a 12-lead ECG before admitting the woman to an appropriate emergency department or centre providing primary percutaneous coronary intervention (PCI).

It must be noted that intermittent episodes of simple arrhythmia (e.g. supraventricular tachycardia or ectopic beats) are common in pregnancy and often symptoms such as palpitations do not cause significant compromise. However, a pre-hospital call to a collapsed woman where the ECG demonstrates an arrhythmia has to be construed as an emergency and should be treated as per normal guidelines and referred for cardiac assessment.

Acute cardiogenic pulmonary oedema occurs rarely during pregnancy and will usually present with typical findings including shortness of breath, increasing nocturnal dyspnea and orthopnoea, and coughing up pink frothy sputum.

> **TOP TIP**
>
> **Aortic dissection should always be considered in pregnant and postpartum women with atypical chest pain (particularly if the pain is interscapular in association with hypertension).**

Pre-hospital management

Pain, acute shortness of breath or any systemic sign or symptom that compromises the patient's haemodynamic status should be considered a pre-hospital emergency. A full ABCDEFG assessment will assist in determining the nature of the problem. Remember that this is potentially a life-threatening emergency for the mother and baby.

Whilst performing an obstetric primary survey and obtaining an obstetric history:

1. Open, maintain and protect the airway in accordance with the patient's clinical need.
2. If oxygen saturation on air falls below 94%, give oxygen. If SpO_2 is less than 85%, use a non-rebreathing mask; otherwise use a simple face mask. Aim for a target saturation of 94–98%.
3. It may be more appropriate in this situation for the patient to sit upright if they are more comfortable in this position.
4. If the patient is experiencing chest pain suggestive of ACS, manage as for a non-obstetric patient: administer 300 mg soluble aspirin to chew and administer glyceryl trinitrate (GTN) spray 400 micrograms sublingually.
5. Assess a full set of baseline observations, including blood glucose level and record a 12-lead ECG.
6. Initiate transfer to the most appropriate hospital according to local guidelines, based on their ECG. If an ST-elevation myocardial infarction has been diagnosed consider taking the patient directly to a unit capable of providing primary PCI.
7. Provide a pre-alert call to the receiving hospital.
8. Insert a large-bore cannula en route (do NOT delay on scene to do this).
9. Provide intravenous morphine for moderate to severe pain with an antiemetic (e.g. cyclizine or ondansetron) if necessary.

> **TOP TIP**
>
> **Pre-hospital thrombolysis is contraindicated in pregnancy.**

10.2 Epilepsy in pregnancy

Definition

This is defined as a continuing tendency to have seizures. Epilepsy manifests itself through a wide range of signs and symptoms. These range from a tremor in one limb through to a whole-body convulsion, or from an unpleasant taste in the patient's mouth to unconsciousness. On average, one person in 170 in the UK is being treated for epilepsy. It is estimated that the risk of premature death within this group is 2–3 times higher than in the general population (Hanna et al., 2002).

Convulsions are predominantly classified as partial or generalised. Partial (focal) convulsions can be further subdivided as simple or complex and it is rare for either to compromise the pre-hospital patient in a way that requires immediate intervention. Generalised convulsions can also be subdivided and are referred to as either an absence or as a tonic-clonic episode. The latter will concern the pre-hospital practitioner in pregnancy as it can be impossible to differentiate from eclampsia. Eight maternal deaths occurred in the UK as a result of epilepsy in the period from 2013 to 2015 (MBRRACE-UK, 2017).

Risk factors

- Poor compliance
- Sleep deprivation
- Hyperemesis
- Stopping anticonvulsant medication during pregnancy
- Unstable epilepsy
- Reduced efficacy of medications through altered pharmacokinetics (caused by changes in absorption or dilution and hyperemesis) in pregnancy, which can exacerbate pre-existing epilepsy

> **TOP TIP**
>
> **Pregnant women with epilepsy often face additional physical, mental health or social problems. As with all women with these types of problems, additional effort should be taken to ensure they have access to the care they need. This should take into account interpersonal dynamics which may be challenging, provide properly trained interpreters where necessary, and link up with agencies outside the health service (including prisons, probation services, police forces and social services).**

Diagnosis

A convulsing patient may or may not have epilepsy. Most patients you are called to will be postictal by the time you arrive. A patient who is convulsing continuously for more than 5 minutes, or who has repeated convulsions without recovering consciousness in between, is considered to be in *status epilepticus*. It should be remembered, however, that a patient who is not known to be epileptic should be managed using eclampsia guidelines (see Chapter 9). Vasovagal attacks are common in pregnancy and may lead to generalised convulsions. However, even if there is a strong suspicion that a convulsion may have resulted from a relatively benign cause, such as a vasovagal episode, the patient will still need a full hospital assessment to exclude eclampsia and other significant pathologies.

Other less common causes of convulsions during pregnancy include:

- Drug or alcohol withdrawal
- Dysrhythmias
- Pseudoepilepsy
- Hypoglycaemia
- Thrombotic thrombocytopenic purpura
- Cerebral infarction
- Hypocalcaemia
- Gestational epilepsy (convulsions confined to pregnancy)
- Meningitis
- Cerebral vein thrombosis

A thorough ABCDEFG assessment may help identify the underlying cause of the convulsion. Getting to the point quickly is essential; this will help pinpoint the cause and the associated treatment, for instance assessing the blood glucose level and the urine for proteinuria.

> **TOP TIP**
>
> **A fitting obstetric patient who is not known to be epileptic should be managed using eclampsia guidelines.**

Pre-hospital management

A convulsing obstetric patient represents a time-critical emergency. Whilst time on scene should be minimised, it is appropriate to stabilise your patient prior to moving her, when conditions allow. It is preferable to attempt to control the convulsion before handling and moving the patient; moving a convulsing obstetric patient is particularly challenging.

1. Manage the ABCs as outlined before.
2. Treat for eclampsia if the patient is not known to have epilepsy (see Chapter 7). Be aware that eclampsia can also occur in a patient who has epilepsy – treat for eclampsia if in any doubt.
3. If the patient is still convulsing, give a benzodiazepine to stop the seizure. Suitable options include diazepam IV/PR (10–20 mg titrated to effect), buccal midazolam (10 mg) or lorazepam IV (up to 4 mg).
4. A blood glucose test should be performed; if the reading is low, the patient should be managed in accordance with the treatment of hypoglycaemia guidelines.
5. If the convulsion cannot be controlled in the pre-hospital environment the patient will need rapid removal to hospital.
6. An obstetric patient who has had a seizure, even if they are known to have epilepsy and have fully recovered, should be transported to hospital for a full assessment, as significant pathologies cannot safely be excluded at the scene.

10.3 Venous thromboembolism in pregnancy

Definition

A venous thromboembolism (VTE) is a thrombus (blood clot) in part of the circulatory system which has the potential to become detached. This clot can then be moved by the blood through the vessels and lodged in another part of the system – the location determining the nature and severity of the symptoms. The thrombus usually originates in the deep veins of the legs or pelvis and is referred to as a deep vein thrombosis (DVT). If it is carried to the pulmonary vasculature it causes a pulmonary embolism (PE). Ileofemoral thrombi are the most common form of DVT and also are more likely to embolise. VTE is estimated to be up to ten times more common in pregnant women than in non-pregnant women of the same age (RCOG, 2001). Thromboembolism in the form of either PE or cerebral venous thrombosis has been found to be the highest direct cause of maternal death in the UK (MBRRACE-UK, 2017). It is predicted that many of these deaths could be avoided with improved recognition of risk factors, greater and earlier appreciation of the signs and symptoms, and earlier implementation of either prophylaxis or treatment.

Risk factors

- Age (particularly over 35 years)
- Obesity (body mass index greater than 30 kg/m² either pre or early pregnancy)
- Parity of four or more
- Family or previous history of thromboembolism
- Gross varicose veins
- Major concurrent illness (e.g. cancer, cardiorespiratory disease, inflammatory bowel disease)
- Prolonged immobility, including more than 4 days of bed rest
- Paraplegia
- Long haul travel; this is not solely confined to air travel and includes prolonged immobility in association with car, bus or rail travel
- Operative delivery; one-half of all deaths from PE followed delivery by caesarean section (MBRRACE-UK, 2015a)
- Instrumental vaginal delivery
- Prolonged labour (greater than 12 hours)
- Surgical procedures in pregnancy or puerperium
- Prolonged time in lithotomy

Diagnosis

The location of the embolism will determine the nature and severity of the signs and symptoms. A DVT manifests as pain, swelling and tenderness in the calf muscle although lower abdominal pain may be the only presenting symptom in ileofemoral DVT.

The most common findings in PE are tachypnoea, dyspnoea, pleuritic chest pain, cough and haemoptysis. Clinical evidence of DVT is rarely found in patients with PE. Tachycardia may be the only sign of a PE, or there may be no abnormal physical signs at all. A massive PE may present with signs of cyanosis, hypotension, sudden collapse or cardiorespiratory arrest.

Local policies should be in place for the investigation of possible VTE once the patient reaches hospital.

> **TOP TIP**
>
> **Although tachypnoea, dyspnoea and leg pain are commonly found in pregnancy they should be investigated in order to exclude VTE.**

> **TOP TIP**
>
> **The risk of VTE is as high in the first trimester as it is in late pregnancy.**

> **TOP TIP**
>
> **If presented with a haemodynamically unstable patient with sudden onset of tachypnoea, dyspnoea, chest pain and tachycardia, a PE should be considered in your differential diagnosis.**

> **TOP TIP**
>
> **The commonest ECG finding in a patient with a PE is sinus tachycardia. However, patients presenting with massive PE may occasionally show the following 'textbook' ECG changes:**
>
> * **S wave in lead I**
> * **Q wave in lead III**
> * **T wave inversion in lead III**

Pre-hospital management

A suspected PE with haemodynamic instability is a time-critical, life-threatening emergency requiring rapid transfer to hospital.

While performing an obstetric primary survey and obtaining an obstetric history also carry out the following:

1. Assess and manage the ABCs as outlined before.
2. Start transportation without delay to the nearest appropriate hospital.
3. Provide a pre-alert message to the receiving hospital unit.
4. Obtain IV access en route.

10.4 Diabetes in pregnancy

Definition

Diabetes is the most common pre-existing medical disorder complicating pregnancy in the UK, with approximately one pregnant woman in every 250 having pre-existing diabetes (CEMACH, 2007c). Patients with pre-existing diabetes may be of Type I or Type II. In maternity care, Type II diabetes is becoming much more common as it is related to obesity; it may present for the first time in pregnancy.

Gestational diabetes is diabetes appearing in pregnancy for the first time and may require diet, metformin or insulin, or a combination of treatments. It resolves after delivery. It is estimated to develop in up to 12% of women (DoH, 2001).

Normoglycaemia (4–8 mmol/l in pregnancy) is the basis of sound pregnancy care. Unfortunately, diabetes becomes more difficult to manage during pregnancy due to changes in physiology and metabolism. As insulin resistance increases due to the effect of placental hormones, insulin requirements often double during pregnancy in Type I diabetes. Recent studies also demonstrate that many women enter pregnancy with poor glycaemic control and half of all diabetic obstetric patients suffer recurrent hypoglycaemia. Severe hypoglycaemia requiring emergency treatment is a relatively common complication of diabetes in pregnancy (CEMACH, 2007c). Diabetic ketoacidosis (DKA) is relatively rare in pregnancy but when it does occur, it requires prompt and skilled management to avert a poor outcome. Fortunately, maternal deaths from diabetes remain rare (CEMACH, 2007a).

Risk factors

- Obesity
- Family history
- Ethnic group – especially if from the Indian subcontinent
- Previous impaired glucose tolerance or gestational diabetes
- Advanced maternal age (more than 40 years)

Diagnosis

De novo (new) diabetes

- Thirst
- Polyuria
- Weight loss
- Persistent heavy glycosuria
- Polyhydramnios
- Increased fetal growth
- Raised random blood sugar
- Features of DKA (see following)

Hypoglycaemia

This may occur with any type of diabetes for which the patient is receiving medication, which may be oral hypoglaemic agents and/or insulin. It does not occur in patients whose diabetes is controlled purely by diet.

- Pallor
- Sweating
- Malaise
- Shaking/shivering
- Blood sugar below 4 mmol/l
- Altered mental state
- Reducing level of consciousness

Diabetic ketoacidosis

This is usually in association with a concurrent illness, infection (a urinary tract infection is common) or poor diabetic control (sometimes due to poor compliance). Note not all symptoms may be present.

- Polyuria
- Polydipsia
- Nausea and vomiting
- Abdominal cramps
- Dehydration
- Shivering
- Hyperglycaemia
- Altered mental state
- Falling level of consciousness
- Dysrhythmia
- Ketotic breath

- Ketonuria
- Raised serum lactate
- Kussmaul's respirations

Pregnancy complications associated with diabetes

Women with either pre-existing diabetes or gestational diabetes are at increased risk of many complications of pregnancy. These include:

- Miscarriage
- Hypertensive disorders
- Abnormalities of fetal growth – babies can be too big or too small
- Stillbirth
- Shoulder dystocia
- Antepartum and postpartum haemorrhage

TOP TIP

Hypoglycaemia and DKA in pregnancy are true medical emergencies requiring assessment and urgent hospital admission.

TOP TIP

The fetus may die as a result of poor glycaemic control. Hospital referral is important in order to check fetal well-being and viability.

Pre-hospital management

Hypoglycaemia

1. Manage the ABCs as outlined before, including a measurement of blood glucose.
2. If the patient is hypoglycaemic and conscious, encourage the consumption of carbohydrates, sugary foods/drinks or glucose gels.
3. If the patient is hypoglycaemic and unconscious, insert a large-bore cannula and administer boluses of 10% glucose in accordance with local guidelines.
4. If IV access is not available, give glucagon 1 mg IM.
5. After regaining consciousness, the patient should be encouraged to eat carbohydrate-rich food so that the blood sugar is maintained.
6. Initiate transfer to the nearest appropriate hospital, according to local guidelines.
7. Consider a pre-alert message to the receiving hospital, particularly if the patient's conscious level remains reduced.

Diabetic ketoacidosis

1. Assess and manage the ABCs as outlined before.
2. In the presence of hyperglycaemia and symptoms suggestive of DKA, do not attempt to gain IV access at scene, but initiate immediate transfer to hospital.
3. Provide a pre-alert message to the hospital.
4. En route, obtain IV access with large-bore cannulae and commence fluid therapy with a 250 ml bolus of saline, repeated to a maximum of 1 litre.
5. Continually monitor the patient's vital signs, with specific attention to the ECG.

10.5 Respiratory disease in pregnancy

Definition

Asthma is the most common respiratory disease in pregnancy, affecting between 4% and 12% of pregnant women (Murphy et al., 2005). The overall tidal volume in pregnancy is decreased, with an increased oxygen demand, and a mother may become breathless more easily. Asthma is associated with bronchospasm, mucosal swelling and excessive mucus production that further reduces ventilatory capacity. The severity of asthma varies, remaining stable in one-third of women, worsening in another third and improving in the remainder (Rey and Boulet, 2007).

Other causes of respiratory problems in pregnancy include tuberculosis (TB), cystic fibrosis and infections. TB is on the increase again in the UK, related to patterns of migration as well as to HIV infection. As care with cases of cystic fibrosis has improved, more women with the disease are now becoming pregnant. These patients are more likely to suffer respiratory compromise, particularly in late pregnancy. A woman with chickenpox (varicella) in pregnancy is at high risk of developing varicella pneumonitis, significant respiratory compromise and adult respiratory distress syndrome (ARDS). Influenza strains occurring in recent pandemics have caused particularly severe illness, and an increased risk of death, in pregnant women. Other infective causes of respiratory problems are treated in the same way as for the non-obstetric patient, except that consideration should be given to transporting them to a hospital with obstetric facilities rather than simply the nearest emergency department when this is safe and feasible.

(See also previous section on pulmonary embolism and Chapter 7 on amniotic fluid embolism.)

Risk factors

- Women with poor asthma control prior to pregnancy
- Women with a history of TB
- Women with other respiratory diseases
- Immigrants from areas with high prevalence of TB
- Obese women
- Smokers
- HIV infection

Diagnosis

Asthma is generally diagnosed and managed in general practice. However, there is evidence to suggest that the preventative management of asthma during pregnancy is still not ideal. The differential diagnoses in pregnant women with dyspnoea will require the pre-hospital practitioner to take a full obstetric history.

> **TOP TIP**
>
> **Rarely, severe pre-eclampsia may present with dyspnoea as the main symptom.**

> **TOP TIP**
>
> **A degree of hyperventilation is normal in early pregnancy. This should not be a concern if the patient is not distressed and there is no suspicion of more serious disease.**

With significant respiratory compromise, the patient will have dyspnoea (worsened on exertion) and tachypnoea. In asthma there will be a reduced peak expiratory flow rate. They may be unable to talk in full sentences and will use accessory muscles. They may adopt a tripod posture to increase ventilation (sitting upright, leaning forwards on their arms).

> **TOP TIP**
>
> **Beware the absence of wheeze in a dyspnoeic asthma patient, who is otherwise deteriorating: this is more likely to represent a significant reduction in air entry, rather than an improvement in their condition.**

Pre-hospital management of asthma exacerbation

The principles for the management of dyspnoea (including asthma) are the same as for non-obstetric patients. Chronic obstructive pulmonary disease is extremely rare in this group and standard high-concentration oxygen can be used in the presence of respiratory compromise. A patient with signs of life-threatening asthma should have airway and breathing treatment initiated before rapidly being transferred to hospital.

While performing an obstetric primary survey and obtaining an obstetric history also carry out the following:

1. Manage the ABCs in the standard way as described earlier. Patients with significant respiratory distress may need to be seated upright, or semi-recumbent in a left lateral tilt.
2. Start transportation immediately to the nearest hospital for life-threatening and severe attacks of asthma.

3. For acute life-threatening and severe exacerbations of asthma, treat en route to hospital (treat on scene for moderate attacks):
   a. Give salbutamol 5 mg via an oxygen-driven continuous nebuliser until symptoms are reversed. Consider using a nebuliser attached to a T-piece and bag–valve–mask in patients requiring ventilatory support.
   b. Add ipratropium bromide 500 micrograms to the first dose of salbutamol for acute life-threatening or severe asthma, or in moderate exacerbations to the second nebuliser if there is no response to the first dose of salbutamol.
   c. Give hydrocortisone 200 mg by slow IV push (consider oral prednisolone 40 mg for moderate and severe attacks).
   d. If available and no response to other drugs, administer a single 2 g dose of magnesium sulphate by IV infusion over 20 minutes.
   e. In extremis, consider adrenaline 500 micrograms IM
   f. Consider crystalloid IV infusion to treat dehydration and limit mucous plugging in patients having a prolonged asthma attack.
4. Transfer to hospital urgently.
5. Pre-alert the receiving hospital if the patient has a severe or life-threatening exacerbation of asthma.
6. Record a full set of baseline observations including peak expiratory flow rate (PEFR) (tables and online resources are available for estimating a patient's predicted PEFR; note that the PEFR may be less than normal in the pregnant woman even in the absence of asthma).

TOP TIP

Due to the physiological changes associated with pregnancy, overall lung capacity is reduced. Peak expiratory flow meter readings may be less than normal as predicted by the patient or a standard chart. However, treat a dyspnoeic and compromised patient regardless of peak expiratory flow.

10.6 Trauma in pregnancy

Definition

The majority of maternal deaths attributed to trauma in the UK occur due to domestic violence and murder in vulnerable and socially excluded women (CEMACH, 2007a). One-third of women who experience domestic violence are hit for the first time whilst pregnant (Duxbury, 2014). Between 2009 and 2013, 13 women were murdered during pregnancy or up to 6 weeks after their pregnancy, with over half of these women killed by stabbing (MBRRACE-UK, 2015a). Deaths caused through road traffic collisions (RTCs) constitute the second largest group.

TOP TIP

All healthcare providers should be aware of the increased risk of domestic violence in pregnancy. This is often directed at the pregnant abdomen and can therefore be linked to placental abruption.

Risk factors

Domestic violence

- Women who are in abusive relationships and/or surrounded by complex social circumstances
- Young and socially excluded women
- Women with children who are the subject of a child protection plan
- Drugs and alcohol abuse

Road traffic collisions

- Women not wearing seatbelts
- Wearing the seatbelt incorrectly – previous reports have highlighted the importance of a correctly worn seatbelt in reducing mortality (CEMACH, 2007d). Consequently, wearing the seatbelt correctly in pregnancy is now actively promoted in an attempt to reduce this trend (Figure 10.1)

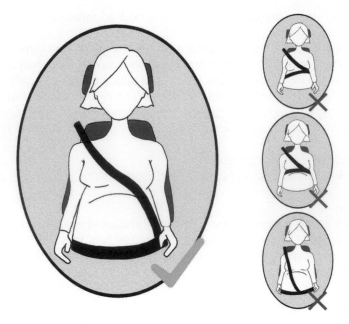

Figure 10.1 Correct and incorrect seatbelt wearing

Diagnosis

The aim is to identify injuries placing the mother and baby at risk. Remember to consider the possibility of placental abruption (see Chapter 9); this may occur several days after the initial incident.

> **TOP TIP**
>
> **In trauma, as in other causes of significant pathology in pregnancy, the cardinal rule of treatment is that resuscitation of the mother facilitates resuscitation of the fetus.**

> **TOP TIP**
>
> **Documenting the precise mechanism of injury (MOI) is imperative in the pre-hospital environment. This may aid assessment of what damage has occurred to internal organs and structures and specifically to the gravid uterus in the third trimester.**

Pre-hospital management

Most simple wounds and superficial burns may be successfully dealt with in the pre-hospital environment. However, obstetric patients with significant blunt or penetrating trauma to the abdomen or elsewhere should be referred to hospital for assessment. A thorough ABCDEFG approach should be applied to patient assessment and ongoing monitoring. The practitioner should specifically assess for fetal movement and also ascertain if the mother is complaining of abdominal pain. The occurrence of vaginal blood loss following a traumatic incident is a 'red flag' and should indicate that the patient is time-critical, until proven otherwise.

The management of the ABCs in an obstetric trauma patient follows a similar pattern to that for a non-trauma patient. However, there are some important modifications that need to be made – these are outlined here.

1. Control any external catastrophic haemorrhage, using direct and indirect pressure or tourniquets where indicated.
2. Manually displace the uterus to the left until the patient can be secured to a spine board and tilted.
3. Provide cervical spine protection as necessary.
4. Secure the patient onto a spine board or scoop and place sufficient padding under the right side of the board to produce a 15–30° tilt.
5. Simultaneously with the above, open, maintain and protect the airway in accordance with the patient's clinical need.

6. Use supplementary oxygen as necessary, aiming for target saturations of 94–98%.
7. Assess the efficacy of the patient's ventilation and provide assistance where indicated (e.g. persistent low saturation, inadequate tidal volume).
8. If the patient has a thoracic injury that affects the mechanism of breathing, the management and intervention must be the same as for a non-obstetric patient.
9. Local guidelines should be followed to decide on the most appropriate disposition, such as to a major trauma centre (MTC), a trauma unit or an emergency department with an associated obstetric unit.
10. Insert one or two large-bore (14 G) cannulae en route (do NOT delay on scene to do this). If it is not possible to gain IV access, consider using an IO cannula.
11. Administer crystalloids in 250 ml aliquots as required to maintain a systolic BP of 90 mmHg.
12. Apply splints to pelvic and long bone fractures.
13. Administer analgesia if the patient is in pain – use morphine cautiously if the patient is hypotensive.
14. Check blood glucose level en route, and treat accordingly.
15. If the patient has been burned assess, treat and manage their burns in exactly the same manner as for a non-obstetric patient. If burns are estimated to be more than 25% body surface area (BSA), give 1 litre of crystalloid IV.
16. If the patient's injuries are non-time-critical, a full secondary survey should be performed, although the need to minimise scene time must be borne in mind.
17. Ensure that the patient is kept as warm as possible before and during transport – if hypothermia occurs, it can contribute to coagulopathy and hence increased bleeding.
18. The use of Tranexamic Acid is recommended in the management of traumatic haemorrhage in pregnancy, as in the non-pregnant patient.

TOP TIP

Even significant hypovolaemia may not result in symptoms in the obstetric patient until 35% of their blood volume is lost.

TOP TIP

Although abdominal and back pains are common in pregnancy, in cases of RTCs and abdominal trauma, a full assessment will be required to exclude significant injury and this must be carried out in the hospital setting. Local guidelines for the most appropriate disposition should be followed.

TOP TIP

Abruption may occur 3 or 4 days after the initial incident and after the patient has been discharged home.

10.7 Substance misuse in pregnancy

Definition

The excessive use of either legal or illegal substances in pregnancy may have effects on fetal viability and growth as well as subsequent development postnatally.

Substance abuse or misuse often involves a mother either continuing to drink alcohol, smoke cannabis, inhale solvent fumes or engaging in the use of illegal drugs such as cocaine, heroin, amphetamines or benzodiazepines. In many situations, the same individual uses more than one of the these substances at a given time. Polysubstance misuse makes a significant contribution to maternal mortality.

Risk factors

- History of previous substance misuse
- Socially excluded (e.g. being homeless or living in very poor circumstances)
- Failure to access antenatal care
- Other children in care or the subject of a child protection plan
- Failure to seek or attend antenatal care

Diagnosis

A mother taking illegal substances during pregnancy increases her risk of anaemia and multiple infections (bacterial endocarditis, cellulitis and blood-borne infections, e.g. hepatitis and HIV.) The incidence of miscarriage, antepartum haemorrhage (in particular placental abruption), growth restriction and preterm labour are significantly increased when the mother has been using cocaine or heroin.

Alcohol misuse can have both fetal and maternal effects. The fetus is at risk of growth restriction and more specifically 'fetal alcohol syndrome'. Both the mother and fetus are at risk of the consequences of trauma secondary to alcohol intoxication.

Growth restriction and antepartum haemorrhage are more common amongst the 17% of pregnant women who continue to smoke during their pregnancy (NHS Digital, 2017). Miscarriage rates are more than 25% higher compared with non-smokers.

Patients who are victims of substance misuse may present with collapse and it is vitally important to exclude other obstetric and non-obstetric causes before making the assumption that collapse is due to intoxication/overdose. A history from witnesses or relatives is vital and patient hand-held records should be reviewed.

Pre-hospital management

The priorities in managing an obstetric patient who is apparently intoxicated are the same as with any adult patient, other than positioning. The specific cause of collapse will dictate how the patient is managed and this is covered in other sections. General principles include:

1. Manage the ABCs in the standard way as described earlier.
2. A full ABCDEFG assessment will assist in deciding the nature of the problem.
3. Ensure the patient is positioned appropriately to reduce aortocaval compression – 15–30° left lateral tilt or manual uterine displacement.
4. Based on the findings of your assessment, treat and manage as indicated. Remember to administer drug-specific antidotes/supportive treatment if appropriate (e.g. naloxone for opiates should be used as in the non-obstetric patient). Initiate transfer to the most appropriate emergency department according to local guidelines.
5. Provide a pre-alert call to the receiving hospital.

10.8 Carbon monoxide poisoning in pregnancy

Definition

Carbon monoxide (CO) occurs in the environment as a result of incomplete combustion of natural or petroleum gas. Haemoglobin has a greater affinity for CO than for oxygen. Consequently, CO molecules in the blood are readily taken up and bound to haemoglobin. This creates carboxyhaemoglobin, which is incapable of carrying oxygen, and in consequence tissue hypoxia can occur. CO is a particularly dangerous gas because it has no taste or smell and it cannot be seen.

Carbon monoxide poisoning in pregnancy is worthy of particular mention because it leads to fetal hypoxia. Firstly, the oxygen content of maternal blood falls as maternal carboxyhaemoglobin levels rise. Secondly, as CO crosses the placenta, it is taken up by the fetal haemoglobin to a greater extent than maternal haemoglobin, reducing the fetal haemoglobin's capacity to deliver oxygen.

Risk factors

About 50 people per year in the UK die at home as a result of CO poisoning through inhalation of trapped gas. Causes include faulty gas boilers and fires (in particular blocked flues and inadequate ventilation), and blocked chimneys in wood and coal burning fires and stoves. Car exhausts are a potent source of CO – fumes can build up rapidly (within minutes) in a closed garage, and whilst this can cause poisoning accidentally, it is also a method used to attempt suicide.

The incidence of CO poisoning is likely to be higher in socially disadvantaged groups because of difficulties in the affordability of regular servicing of heating equipment.

Diagnosis

Mild CO poisoning may be misdiagnosed by the sufferer or healthcare professionals as a cold or flu. Symptoms may include headache, nausea, dizziness, sore throat and a cough. If it occurs as a result of a faulty household appliance, it is almost certain that all family members and residents living in the accommodation will be affected – but this may increase the likelihood of a misdiagnosis being made of an infective cause.

Moderate poisoning may result in additional symptoms such as confusion, loss of memory and poor coordination.

Severe CO poisoning will cause tachycardia, arrhythmias, hyperventilation and/or dyspnoea, an altered mental status or reduced level of consciousness and convulsions. If untreated, death will ensue. The symptoms of moderate to severe CO poisoning may be misdiagnosed as having a cardiac, neurological or respiratory aetiology.

A differential diagnosis should be made based on the environmental evidence. Have a high index of suspicion if presented with a patient (or patients living together) with the above constellation of symptoms. As faulty heating appliances are the most common cause of CO poisoning at home, be particularly aware of this risk during cold weather when heaters have been used for prolonged periods, particularly if this occurs immediately after a warm spell or at the end of summer. If possible, ask when gas appliances were last serviced or chimneys swept.

The fire service carries CO detectors and consequently should be asked to attend any suspicious incident to assist in confirming the diagnosis.

Pulse oximetry is likely to be unreliable in CO poisoning, as most devices currently on the market are unable to distinguish between oxyhaemoglobin and carboxyhaemoglobin as they detect only two wavelengths of light. Consequently, the percentage of haemoglobin that is actually saturated with oxygen will be lower than that indicated by the SpO_2 monitor. Some newer monitors have the capability to measure up to seven wavelengths and this enables them to accurately distinguish between oxyhaemoglobin and carboxyhaemoglobin and to give measurements for both.

> **TOP TIP**
>
> **Remember that if the mother has CO poisoning, so will the fetus.**

> **TOP TIP**
>
> **The readings obtained by most pulse oximeters are unreliable in CO poisoning: the reading provided will be falsely high and tends towards 100% regardless of the true percentage of haemoglobin saturated with oxygen. Remember the true percentage of oxygen-saturated haemoglobin will be lower than that indicated by the SpO_2 monitor.**

Pre-hospital management

1. Consider your own safety above all else. Do NOT enter non-respirable atmospheres without appropriate equipment. If rescue is necessary, this should be performed by the fire service using self-contained breathing apparatus. If you inadvertently enter an environment contaminated with CO your only warning may be the onset of symptoms as described. If this occurs, LEAVE THE SCENE IMMEDIATELY and seek fresh air.
2. Arrange for urgent removal of the casualties from the contaminated environment – those with mild to moderate symptoms should be able to self-evacuate. Open windows and outside doors to allow a flow of fresh air to facilitate this.
3. Remember to place recumbent pregnant patients in either the left lateral position or tilted 15–30° to the left.
4. If necessary, secure and protect the airway; consider early intubation in severely obtunded obstetric patients.
5. If the patient is conscious, provide as high a concentration of oxygen as possible, using a tightly fitted non-rebreathing mask. If the patient is unconscious and has a respiratory rate of <10 or >30 breathes per minute, consider assisting ventilations with a self-inflating bag with an oxygen reservoir and high-concentration oxygen or a mechanical ventilator set for 100% oxygen.
6. As soon as airway access and ventilatory support have been facilitated, rapidly transfer to the nearest emergency department.
7. Provide a pre-alert message en route to the hospital.
8. Obtain IV access en route to the hospital.
9. Be aware that the patient may require urgent transfer to a facility with a hyperbaric chamber.

> **TOP TIP**
>
> **The mainstay of treatment for CO poisoning is delivery of oxygen, at as high a concentration as possible. Treating the mother will treat the fetus.**

10.9 Rape and sexual assault in pregnancy

Definition

Rape is defined by the Sexual Offences Act 2003 as penetration by a penis of the vagina, anus or mouth of another person without their consent. 'Consent' in the context of the offence of rape is now defined in the Act. A person can be said to have consented if he or she agrees by choice, and has the freedom and capacity to make that choice. The law does not require the victim to have resisted physically. The defendant must also show that his belief in the consent of the person was reasonable. In deciding whether this belief was reasonable, a jury must consider any steps the defendant took to confirm that the person was consenting to sexual activity. If the victim was unconscious, drugged, abducted or subject to threats or fear of serious harm, it will be presumed that the victim could not consent to the sexual activity and that the defendant could not have reasonably believed that the victim consented. The definition of sexual assault is similar to that of rape as the intentional sexual penetration of the vagina or anus of another person with a part of their body or anything else, where the recipient does not consent to the penetration, and the defendant cannot show a reasonable belief that consent existed (CPS, 2009).

Risk factors

Many people believe that the majority of cases of rape involve an attack on a woman by a male aggressor who is unknown to her. In reality, the majority of rape victims know their attacker. A married woman can be raped by her husband, and rape can also occur in the context of other established relationships. Many victims of sexual assault – perhaps the majority – do not report the offence to the police.

Diagnosis

Diagnosis should be on the basis of history. However, rape victims may be reluctant to discuss what has happened to them, perhaps because of a misplaced belief that they are in some way to blame. Consequently, pre-hospital providers must be alert to circumstantial evidence that suggests the patient may be a victim of a sexual assault. Stories of how injuries have occurred that do not match the normal mechanism of injuries found, torn clothing, a reluctance to be examined and concerns about being left alone with male practitioners, friends or family may all occur in the context of rape. Ultimately, the wishes of the patient must be respected, and if they do not wish to report the crime then the healthcare worker cannot overrule this. You should, however, tactfully try to determine the true cause of any injuries found in order that all appropriate treatment may be offered, including psychological support.

Rape is a very traumatic event. The patient may present as being confused; they may be crying, nervous and fearful, or laughing inappropriately; they may be hostile towards healthcare practitioners, or they may appear numb and withdrawn. Victims may delay calling for assistance, and may shower or change their clothes before doing so. In addition to psychological sequelae, signs and symptoms in pregnant rape victims may include trauma to the vagina or anus, or more general injuries resulting from the assault. Vaginal bleeding may occur subsequent to local trauma, a placenta praevia or (rarely) an abruption. Any physical examination should be limited to that necessary to find and treat serious injuries. The patient's consent to an examination should always be sought and their wishes respected.

Pre-hospital management

1. Manage the ABCs as necessary and in accordance with any injuries or illnesses found.
2. The same healthcare provider should stay with the patient until handover at the hospital, once a rapport has been established. In the absence of significant physical injuries, emotional support is the most valuable intervention that pre-hospital providers can provide.
3. Although, with the patient's permission, the police should be contacted immediately, the patient should be taken to an appropriate emergency department rather than a police station. If called to the scene, the police may wish to accompany the patient in the ambulance – again this must be with the patient's agreement.

4. Remember that a crime has taken place. Local services that provide forensic examination, such as sexual assault referral centres (SARCs), should be contacted if advice is required. Even if the victim initially refuses to involve the police, try to avoid the loss of any evidence as the patient may change their mind. Healthcare professionals should only remove as much clothing as is necessary to safely examine the patient, and should document any damage that they have caused to clothing in doing so (e.g. cutting off clothes to permit access to a serious injury). Clothing should be retained in paper bags, rather than plastic, as this allows better preservation of DNA evidence.

5. Carefully document any signs of trauma and any information about the circumstances of the attack that the victim shares with you. Both may be required as evidence should the victim decide to involve the police.

6. As well as treating any specific injuries or obstetric or gynaecological problems, hospital treatment will need to address the probability of the patient suffering a sexually transmitted disease. This should include a specific risk assessment for HIV, hepatitis B and hepatitis C exposure. This will allow appropriate provision of prophylactic medication as well as planning and providing psychological support. In many areas, forensic examination and counselling will not take place in the hospital setting but the patient will instead be referred to a SARC or similar facility for these purposes.

10.10 Perinatal psychiatric illness

Definition

Mental illness experienced either during pregnancy or in the postnatal period can affect not only the health and well-being of the mother and baby, but also those providing the usual support network around her. Mental disorders may be pre-existing or develop during pregnancy, the puerperium and up to 1 year after the birth. Depression and anxiety are the most common mental health problems during pregnancy, with around 12% of woman experiencing depression and 13% experiencing anxiety at some point (NICE, 2014). Practitioners should note that the term 'postnatal depression' is often used inappropriately as a general term for any perinatal mental disorder and this should be avoided.

Developing a new onset of serious psychiatric illness during pregnancy is generally thought to be less of a risk than at other times, although the prevalence of all psychiatric disorders such as schizophrenia is the same in either pregnant or non-pregnant women. Between 2009 and 2013 there were 161 maternal deaths in the UK as a result of mental health-related causes during or up to 1 year after the end of pregnancy (MBRRACE-UK, 2015a). Pregnancy itself may have a protective effect on the mother, with occurrences of serious mental disorder and suicide occurring predominantly after the birth. The most common method used by women who died by suicide was hanging. All time periods after childbirth pose a greater risk for suicide, when compared with the 9-month antenatal period (MBRRACE-UK, 2015a). According to the 2013–15 MBRRACE-UK report, 14% of all recorded deaths amongst women who died between 6 weeks and 1 year after the end of pregnancy were due to suicide (MBRRACE-UK, 2017).

Risk factors

- Women in late pregnancy and the first 3 months' postpartum
- Previous mental health problems
- Family history of serious mental illness, including schizophrenia, bipolar and postnatal psychosis
- Social isolation, especially if the baby has been removed by social services
- History of domestic abuse
- Previous puerperal psychosis
- Recent termination
- Unwanted pregnancy

Diagnosis

The pre-hospital diagnosis of psychiatric illness is difficult. Expert evaluation is always necessary. The signs and symptoms associated with psychoses or neuroses will be the same in the obstetric patient as they are for any other patient. The method of suicide chosen by pregnant women is, however, predominantly violent in nature.

A thorough physical examination is necessary to exclude any physical cause for symptoms.

Pre-hospital management

Newly presenting psychiatric symptoms may require specific treatment such as counselling or medication. Counselling services can be difficult to access in the pre-hospital environment. Admission and referral may be required, but consideration should also be given to accessing primary care services.

In patients presenting with a mental disorder that is affecting their health and well-being, the priority will be to provide support and guidance, not only for them but also for other family members.

It is important to assess whether the patient has the capacity to make decisions. Pre-hospital practitioners need to ensure that they are familiar with guidance on gaining consent to examine or treat their patients, and the focus is on the needs of the mother. If the patient refuses admission and lacks capacity they should be urgently referred to their GP (or out-of-hours service) for consideration for sectioning under the Mental Health Act. Pre-hospital practitioners will have to await the arrival of other healthcare providers before they can leave the patient.

Referral and transfer to a facility that can provide expert evaluation is the key to the management of significant psychiatric illness. Pre-hospital practitioners will need to rely on the effectiveness of their communication skills to manage these patients appropriately.

Where suicide has been attempted, the treatment and transport criteria will be the same as for any obstetric patient. Differences in treatment approaches from non-obstetric patients after attempted suicide by violent means are as described in Section 10.6.

> **TOP TIP**
>
> **Treating the mother is the best way to treat the baby.**

Summary of key points

- The general principles of ABC management are the same for obstetric patients as for other patients – other than the vital importance of left lateral positioning
- Maternal deaths from cardiac diseases account for more cases than all other causes together. In particular, acute coronary syndrome must be considered in women who are obese and/or heavy smokers
- Poor medication compliance accounts for many epileptic patients suffering fits during pregnancy. Eclampsia should always be considered as a possible cause
- Suspect a pulmonary embolism if presented with a patient with a sudden, unexplained onset of tachypnoea, dyspnoea, chest pain and tachycardia who is hypotensive
- Good diabetic control becomes more difficult to achieve during pregnancy. This may be due to pregnancy physiology or poor concordance (compliance)
- The severity of asthma varies, remaining stable in one-third of women, worsening in another third and improving in the remainder
- In trauma, overt signs of major haemorrhage may not be revealed until the mother has lost approaching 35% of her circulating blood volume
- The misuse of legal and illegal substances during pregnancy can have multiple adverse effects on both the mother and fetus
- Most incidences of acute mental disorder and suicide occur in the last trimester of pregnancy and in the first 90 days following delivery

CHAPTER 11
Normal labour and delivery

Learning outcomes

After reading this chapter, you will be able to:
- Describe the anatomy of the female pelvis
- Explain the mechanism of normal delivery
- Recognise and describe the three stages of labour

11.1 Normal labour and delivery

Anatomy of the female pelvis

The female pelvis is generally wider and broader than that of males, with a more pronounced oval-shaped inlet (Figure 11.1). This 'gynaecoid' pelvis is ultimately different to accommodate the process of childbirth. In obstetric terms, the female pelvis is considered as two regions: the superior section is referred to as the greater or 'false' pelvis. It has limited obstetric relevance but provides support for the lower abdominal viscera. Intuitively, the inferior section is known as the lesser or 'true' pelvis, which contains the pelvic cavity and pelvic viscera.

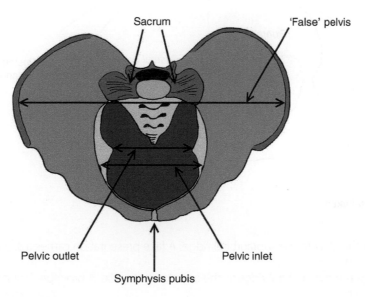

Figure 11.1 Anatomy of the female pelvis

Pre-Obstetric Emergency Training: A Practical Approach, Second Edition. Edited by Mark Woolcock.
© 2019 John Wiley & Sons Ltd. Published 2019 by John Wiley & Sons Ltd.

Pelvic inlet

The junction between the greater and lesser pelvis is known as the **pelvic inlet**. The outer bony edges of the pelvic inlet are called the **pelvic brim**. This is the superior margin of the pelvic cavity and is bounded by the sacral promontory posteriorly, laterally by the iliopectineal lines, and anteriorly by the symphysis pubis. The pelvic inlet determines the size and shape of the birth canal. Significantly, the transverse diameter tends to be greater than the anteroposterior (AP) diameter.

Pelvic cavity

The pelvic cavity has a curved shape because of the difference in size between the anterior and posterior borders of the space created by the pelvic bones. Roughly circular in shape with the transverse and AP diameters tending to be similar, it is bounded by the sacrum posteriorly, laterally by the pubic bone and the obturator fascia and the inner aspect of the ischial bone, and anteriorly by the symphysis pubis. The cavity is referred to as the pelvic canal and is the bony passage through which the baby must pass.

Pelvic outlet

This is the narrowest bony part of the pelvis for the baby to pass through and marks the inferior margin of the pelvic cavity. It is bounded posteriorly by the coccyx, laterally by the ischial tuberosities, and anteriorly by the pubic arch. In regard to the mechanism of normal delivery it is important to note that now the AP diameter tends to be greater than the transverse diameter.

11.2 Fetal skull

Figure 11.2 identifies of certain regions and landmarks of the fetal skull. These have particular importance for obstetric care because they may indicate the **presenting part** of the fetus.

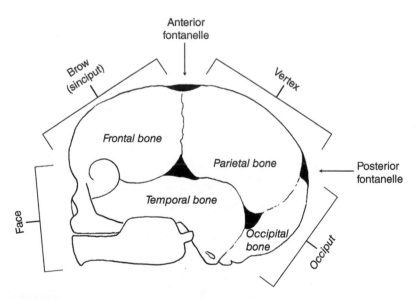

Figure 11.2 Anatomy of the fetal skull

- The **face** extends from the chin to the supraorbital ridge. A face presentation carries a significant risk for both mother and baby (see Chapter 12)
- The **brow** extends from the supraorbital ridge to the anterior fontanelle. A brow presentation also carries a significant risk for both mother and baby
- The **vertex** is the area midway between the anterior fontanelle, the two parietal bones and the posterior fontanelle. A **vertex presentation** occurs when this part of the fetal skull is leading the way. This represents a normal presentation for a vaginal delivery
- The **occiput** is the area between the posterior fontanelle and the base of the skull. It is a very unusual presenting part, carrying a significant risk to mother and baby

Additionally, the following terms are also used as **reference points**: the **sinciput refers to the front of the head** whilst the **occiput refers to the back of the head** and the **mentum refers to the chin**.

The fetal skull bones are as follows:

- The *frontal bone*: the fetal frontal bone consists of two halves that after the age of 8 years fuse to form a single bone
- The two *parietal bones* lie on either side, forming the majority of the skull
- The two *temporal bones,* one on each side of the head, are closest to the ears
- The *occipital bone* forms the back and part of the base of the skull

Sutures are joints between the bones of the skull that permit gliding of one bone over another during moulding of the head. In a vertex presentation the diameter of the head can be reduced to allow easier passage through the birth canal. The sutures begin to harden during childhood, inhibiting movement. This continues into early adulthood until the growing process completes. There are two key landmarks created where the sutures meet, and these are referred to as the fontanelles:

- The **anterior fontanelle** (also known as the bregma) is a diamond-shaped space towards the front of the baby's head. It is formed by four bones, at the junction of the sagittal, coronal and frontal sutures
- The **posterior fontanelle** (or lambda) has a triangular shape, and is found towards the back of the fetal skull. It is formed by three bones at the junction of the lambdoid and sagittal sutures

11.3 Stages of labour

The process of labour is normally divided into three stages as this makes it easier to describe the progress a mother is making. These are explained below.

A very fast labour with a duration of less than 1 hour is referred to as a 'precipitate labour'.

The amniotic membranes and fluid surround the fetus, protecting it within a sterile environment against ascending bacterial infection.

- The membranes can rupture at any point before or during labour
- The amniotic fluid or liquor should be clear and odourless
- If the liquor is bloodstained, this could indicate an abruption or placenta praevia
- If the liquor is yellow or green coloured, this could indicate the presence of meconium and may be an indicator of fetal compromise
- The presence of thick meconium that may contain particulate material is a particular cause for concern

---

TOP TIP

Always consider whether fluid loss could be urine rather than liquor.

11.4 First stage of labour

The first stage can be further divided into the 'latent' and the 'active' phases.

Latent phase of labour

This phase of labour can be experienced for several weeks prior to the onset of active labour. Uterine contractions experienced during this phase cause the cervix to thin and soften before it can start to dilate. Contractions are often irregular with a stop/start pattern without becoming stronger or longer. This is normal.

Active phase of labour

- This is defined as regular uterine contractions causing both cervical effacement and dilatation from 0 to 10 cm
- The presence of a mucus show, which may be bloodstained, is common during both the latent and active first stages of labour and is an indicator of cervical effacement and/or dilatation

- Contractions should increase in length, strength and frequency as the first stage progresses
- The frequency of contractions should be measured over a 10-minute period
- In established labour, there are 3–4 contractions in 10 minutes each of which should last for about 1 minute
- More than five contractions within a 10-minute period can indicate overstimulation and may suggest placental abruption (see Chapter 9)
- The duration of the first stage can range from minutes to several hours

> **TOP TIP**
>
> **Unless absolutely critical, the use of internal vaginal examination should be reserved for those formally trained in assessing cervical dilatation.**

> **TOP TIP**
>
> **The first stage of labour is often faster in second and subsequent pregnancies.**

11.5 Second stage of labour

- The second stage starts once the cervix is fully dilated (10 cm)
- Contractions become more expulsive in nature
- Women may have a strong urge to push; this may be a very similar feeling to opening the bowels and is due to the fetal head pressing against the nerves of the pelvic floor muscles and rectum
- The vertex may be visible at the introitus. In a situation where no midwife is present, this will be the only way of confirming that the second stage is under way
- There is dilatation and gaping of the anus due to deep engagement of the presenting part
- The second stage is completed by delivery of the baby (see Section 11.6 for the mechanism of normal delivery)

> **TOP TIP**
>
> **Occasionally, membranes will be visible at the vaginal entrance but the presenting part will be much higher and the cervix may not be fully dilated. Do not manually rupture the membranes as this may allow the cord to prolapse.**

11.6 Normal mechanism of labour

The mechanism of labour is the passive way in which the fetus makes its way through the birth canal. The movements allow the fetus to negotiate the changing dimensions of the pelvis. As noted, the widest diameter of the pelvic inlet is the transverse dimension, whereas the widest diameter of the outlet is the AP dimension. Thus the widest part of the fetal head enters the pelvis in the transverse dimension and then rotates to emerge in the AP dimension at the outlet. The shoulders similarly follow the rotation.

The commonest presentation is the vertex, and the commonest positions are either left or right occipitoanterior. The lie will be longitudinal and the attitude one of flexion. The engaging diameter of the fetal head is therefore the suboccipito-bregmatic.

Descent

Descent often starts before labour, as the fetal head becomes engaged in the pelvis. In the multigravid woman, engagement may not occur until labour commences. Further descent through the pelvis occurs during labour.

Flexion

When labour starts the head will be in an attitude of natural flexion. This is increased during labour for two reasons:

- Any ovoid object being passed through a tube tends to adapt its long axis to the long axis of the tube
- Head lever – the occipitospinal joint is nearer to the occiput than the sinciput. When the uterus contracts and pressure is applied to the fetal breech, the direction of push naturally flexes the head

Internal rotation

As labour continues the fetal head meets the resistance of the pelvic floor and the occiput rotates forwards from the occipitotransverse or occipitoanterior position to lie under the suprapubic arch, with the sagittal suture lying in the AP diameter (Figure 11.3). The rotation occurs because, in addition to the well-flexed head, the sloping gutter shape of the levatores ani (pelvic muscles) directs the occiput (which is leading) anteriorly.

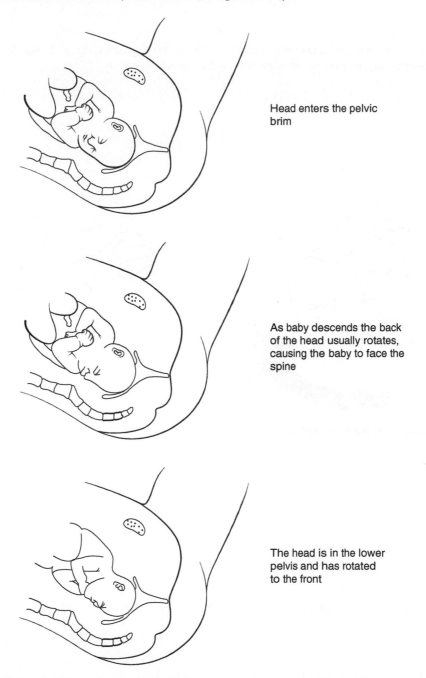

Head enters the pelvic brim

As baby descends the back of the head usually rotates, causing the baby to face the spine

The head is in the lower pelvis and has rotated to the front

Figure 11.3 Internal rotation

The head will then appear at the introitus. The practitioner can control head delivery by gentle pressure.

Crowning

The fetal head has crowned when it emerges from under the pubic arch and no longer recedes between contractions. It will be visible at the introitus.

Encouraging the woman to pant/breathe through the contraction at this stage will help control the delivery of the head.

Extension

The head then delivers by extension (Figure 11.4a). Once the occiput has passed below the symphysis pubis, the head extends with the nape of the neck pressed firmly against the pubic arch. As extension continues the forehead, face and chin deliver over the perineum. It is not necessary to check for the cord as usually the body will deliver through any loops of cord: **clamping and cutting of the cord at this stage is discouraged**.

Restitution

As internal rotation occurs, the fetal head becomes twisted a little on the shoulders (Figure 11.4b). As soon as it is delivered it resumes its natural position with respect to the shoulders. This is called restitution.

(a)   (b)

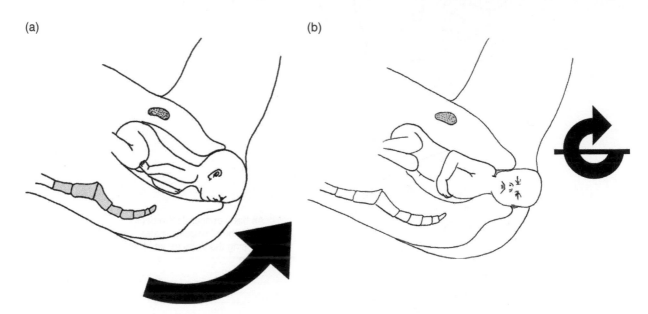

Figure 11.4 (a) Extension and (b) internal rotation

External rotation

At delivery of the head, the shoulders lie in the oblique. With continued descent they rotate to bring the bisacromial diameter into the AP diameter of the pelvic outlet. Rotation of the shoulders occurs as the right and anterior shoulder is lower than the left in the pelvis and meets the resistance of the pelvic floor before the left; it therefore rotates to the space in the front. This causes the head to rotate so that the occiput lies next to the maternal left thigh. This is external rotation. If the fetus is lying the other way around this description should be reversed. External rotation of the head therefore indicates internal rotation of the shoulders.

Delivery of the body

Gentle traction should be applied with hands applied either side of the fetal head, along the line of the long axis of the baby. This is referred to as axial traction (Figure 11.5).

Care should be taken not to apply lateral traction downwards towards the floor, which can result in obstetric brachial plexus injury (OBPI). The anterior shoulder should deliver as the mother pushes.

The direction of axial traction changes to a gentle upward curve after the posterior shoulder appears, and the rest of the body should easily follow (Figure 11.6). Pass the baby up to the mother and ensure skin-to-skin contact to maintain warmth, or resuscitate as necessary.

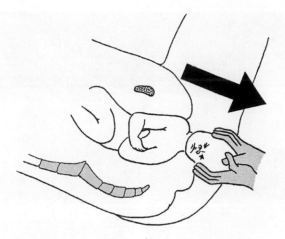

Figure 11.5 Axial traction

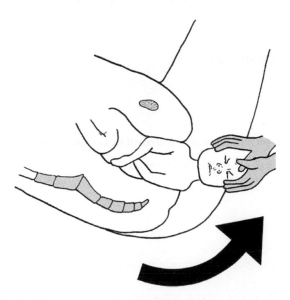

Figure 11.6 Change in direction of axial traction

> **TOP TIP**
>
> **Most babies, if left to their own devices, will deliver spontaneously without any assistance.**

> **TOP TIP**
>
> **Pulling too hard on the baby at delivery can cause a brachial plexus injury.**

Clamping and cutting the umbilical cord

The clamping and cutting of the umbilical cord should be delayed for a minimum of 30–60 seconds following delivery. The baby should be held at or below the level of the placenta during this time to allow the baby to receive an optimum blood volume (ACOG, 2012).

To clamp the cord, place one cord clamp 10–15 cm from the baby's abdomen and a second clamp 2–3 cm distally to the first. Ensure that they are firmly closed and cut between the two clamps (Figure 11.7). The longer length of cord allows venous access at the hospital if required. It may be shortened once a midwife or paediatrician has checked the baby.

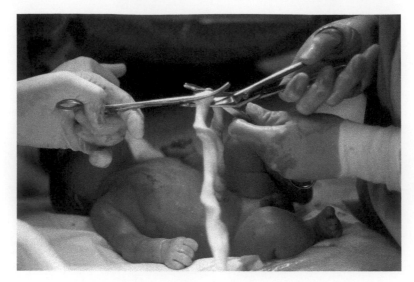

Figure 11.7 Cutting the cord

If the cord snaps immediately, hold and clamp both ends.

TOP TIP

Ensure when cutting the cord, that the baby's fingers and genitals are clear of the scissors.

Ensure that you are cutting between the two clamps (Figure 11.7).

11.7 Third stage

This begins after delivery of the baby and is completed with delivery of the placenta and membranes.

If the placenta stays in situ for more than 30 minutes after an active second stage, it is considered to be retained. A period of 60 minutes can be allowed if a physiological second stage is anticipated – that is, a second stage occuring without the use of uterotonic drugs, no cutting or clamping of the cord until the cord has stopped pulsating, and delivery of the placenta by maternal effort.

The uterus should not be massaged in order to expedite delivery of the placenta as this may result in partial separation. If the placenta partially separates, bleeding can be torrential and urgent action is required – see Chapter 13.

Delivery of the placenta

- Await spontaneous separation of the placenta
- Signs of separation are:
  - Contractions return
  - Cord lengthens
  - Uterus rises up – on abdominal palpation it is easier to feel
  - Often there is a small gush of blood
  - Mother has an urge to push

TOP TIP

Pulling on the cord in an uncontrolled manner may snap the cord or cause a uterine inversion. Therefore this procedure should be performed by only those skilled in obstetrics or midwifery.

> **TOP TIP**
>
> **In the case of twins or higher multiples ensure all babies are delivered before giving an oxytocic agent.**

> **TOP TIP**
>
> **Should the placenta be retained, ensure that the baby has been separated from the umbilical cord by clamping and cutting the cord prior to transfer to hospital.**

Pain relief

Entonox® is an excellent analgesic agent in labour. It is best used starting from the commencement of the pain and throughout the painful period. Deep breaths should be used. Morphine may be required if the woman is extremely distressed with labour pains (10–20 mg IM). However, be aware that the baby may show signs of respiratory depression at delivery.

Emergency care of delivery in the absence of a midwife

- Request the attendance of a midwife to scene and/or additional crew. Direct contact with the maternity department will ensure effective communication and support
- Prepare an area for resuscitation of the baby should it be needed post delivery
- Allow the mother to assume a position of comfort. Do not lay the mother completely flat on her back – upright, propped up or on one side is a much better position
- Prepare a clean, warm area on which to deliver the baby and ensure the availability of warm towels/blankets/hat for the baby
- Make a quick assessment of key events (timing should be noted using the 24-hour clock):
  - Gestation (full term/preterm/non-viable)
  - Number of babies (singleton or multiple pregnancy)
  - Parity of woman (number of previous deliveries)
  - Frequency of contractions over a 10-minute period
  - Urge to push
  - Evidence of bleeding
  - Evidence/time of rupture of membranes
  - Colour of liquor (clear or meconium stained)
  - Is the presenting part visible/advancing during a contraction?
  - Is the head or buttocks presenting? (See Chapter 12, Section 12.3)
- **REASSURE THE MOTHER AT ALL STAGES**
- The baby should be allowed to deliver spontaneously; however, the mother should be encouraged to deliver the head slowly to avoid perineal trauma
- Look for signs of external rotation of the head during the next contraction, which will indicate internal rotation of the shoulders
- If there is delay in delivery of the shoulders, the protocol for shoulder dystocia should be immediately instigated (see Chapter 12, Section 12.10).
- Deliver the baby onto the mother's abdomen and dry/stimulate with a dry towel
- Make a quick assessment of the baby and allow delayed cord clamping for a minimum of 60 seconds as appropriate
- Place the baby skin to skin with the mother and cover with a dry towel/blanket; put on a hat to avoid heat loss
- Document time of delivery of both the head and the body.
- If the baby does not breathe spontaneously or remains blue or white, instigate the neonatal resuscitation procedure (see Chapter 14)
- The umbilical cord should be clamped and cut once it has ceased pulsating or at 5 minutes
- Watch for signs of placental separation:
  - Contractions return (period-type cramps felt)
  - Trickle of blood
  - Cord lengthening
  - Urge to push

- **Allow the placenta to deliver with maternal effort only – DO NOT PULL ON THE CORD**
- Retain the placenta for inspection
- Note blood loss and record amount (<500 or >500 ml)
- If bleeding continues, the protocol for post-partum haemorrhage should be instigated (see Chapter 13, Section 13.1)
- Respiratory rate, pulse and initial blood pressure checks should be performed, but in the absence of bleeding or signs of hypertension or shock no further monitoring is required for the first hour, by which time transfer will usually have been achieved
- Complete separate patient reports for the mother and the baby

---

Summary of key points

- Labour is often faster in second and subsequent pregnancies
- Always consider whether fluid loss could be urine rather than liquor
- Occasionally, membranes will be visible at the vaginal entrance but the presenting part will be much higher and the cervix may not be fully dilated
- Most babies if left to their own devices will deliver spontaneously without any assistance
- Pulling too hard on the baby at delivery can cause a brachial plexus injury
- Allow a minimum of 30–60 seconds delay before clamping and cutting the umbilical cord
- Ensure when cutting the cord, that the baby's fingers and genitals are clear of the scissors
- Ensure that you are cutting between the two clamps and that one clamp is proximal to the baby and the other is more proximal to the placenta.
- Pulling on the cord in an uncontrolled manner may snap the cord or cause a uterine inversion. Therefore, this procedure should only be performed by midwives or obstetricians
- In the case of suspected or known twins or higher multiples ensure all babies are delivered before giving an oxytocic agent. The presence of twins should be anticipated in the absence of an ultrasound scan if the fundal height is greater than expected following delivery
- Ensure that the baby has been separated from the umbilical cord by clamping and cutting the cord prior to transfer to hospital

CHAPTER 12
Complicated labour and delivery

Learning outcomes

After reading this chapter, you will be able to:
- Recognise and describe the management of complications in the first, second and third stages of labour
- Define, identify and describe the pre-hospital management of:
  - Preterm labour
  - Abnormal presentations and lies
  - Multiple pregnancy
  - Shoulder dystocia
  - Umbilical cord problems, including cord prolapse, cord rupture and short cord

---

12.1 Preterm labour

Definition

Preterm labour is defined as labour occurring more than 3 weeks before the expected date of delivery – that is, before the completion of 37 weeks of pregnancy. Preterm labour is a significant predictor of neonatal morbidity and mortality. The survival of newborns delivered before the 24th week of pregnancy is unusual, although not impossible. In 2013, 66% of babies born between 24 and 27 weeks' gestation survived the first 28 days of life, increasing to 89% between 28 and 31 weeks' gestation and 98% at 32–36 weeks' gestation (MBRRACE-UK, 2015b).

Risk factors

- Previous preterm birth
- Twins or higher multiples
- Smoking
- Low socioeconomic groups
- Previous treatment to the cervix
- Known preterm rupture of membranes in the current pregnancy

---

Pre-Obstetric Emergency Training: A Practical Approach, Second Edition. Edited by Mark Woolcock.
© 2019 John Wiley & Sons Ltd. Published 2019 by John Wiley & Sons Ltd.

Diagnosis

The signs and symptoms may be similar to that of normal labour, although there may be little or no contraction pain and the membranes may rupture before the onset of labour. Malpresentations – such as breech presentation – are common. It is unlikely that the head has engaged before labour starts, and if the membranes have ruptured, the practitioner should be aware of the possibility of cord prolapse.

TOP TIP

Preterm labour can proceed rapidly to delivery: a careful assessment may prevent the need to deliver in the back of an ambulance. Abnormal presentations and prolapsed cord are more common than with term labour.

- Assess the patient using the ABCDEFG approach and obstetric primary survey
- Assess the fundal height – remember, if the fundus is below the umbilicus this is equivalent to a pregnancy of less than 20 weeks' gestation, and the fetus is unlikely to be viable
- In particular, remember to get to the point quickly and attempt to identify time-critical problems:
  - Abnormal presentation
  - Prolapsed cord
  - Maternal haemorrhage
- Determine if birth appears to be imminent as this will affect your management plan, and as always obtain an obstetric history from the mother and her patient-held records

Pre-hospital management

1. If your assessment indicates that you can guarantee arriving at the hospital before delivery, commence transportation without delay as a time-critical transfer. Remember to provide the receiving hospital with a pre-alert message.
2. DO NOT commence transportation if the birth appears to be imminent or you assess that it will occur before your arrival at the hospital:
3. Request the attendance of a midwife at the scene.
4. Request the attendance of a second ambulance to provide additional personnel, allowing separate management of the mother and baby after delivery and, if necessary, separate transportation. Ideally, and if time and resources permit, this second ambulance should bring an incubator, but obtaining this should not be permitted to significantly delay its arrival at the incident.
5. Remember you will have two patients, so you will need maternity and paediatric (neonatal) kits, oxygen and Entonox®. Make sure all appropriate kit is available and laid out – prepare a separate area for management of the baby, avoiding draughts if possible.
6. The probability of needing to provide ventilatory or circulatory support to the preterm baby is also higher than with a term delivery.
7. Manage delivery as you would for term labour (see Chapter 11), but be prepared for abnormal presentations and cord prolapse.
8. Maintaining the temperature of the newly born preterm baby is essential. Hypothermia can occur rapidly and is associated with significant morbidity. Remember to dry the baby vigorously and wrap them in clean towels and ensure the head is covered. Only the face should remain exposed. Almost all resuscitative measures can and should be performed without the need to expose the newborn.
9. Carefully assess the baby in accordance with standard procedures. If resuscitation is necessary, follow the guidelines for newborn life support (see Chapter 14).

TOP TIP

In an out-of-hospital environment, if you decide not to move the obstetric patient, request the attendance of a second ambulance *immediately* and at the same time as you request the attendance of a midwife. This will provide additional resources to permit separate care and transportation of the mother and baby.

TOP TIP

Ensure that appropriate measures are taken to ensure the baby is kept warm *immediately* they are born and before resuscitation interventions are undertaken. Cardiopulmonary resuscitation (CPR) and ALS will be ineffective if the baby is allowed to become hypothermic, and this is a particular risk in the pre-hospital setting.

> **TOP TIP**
>
> **Ensure that you monitor both mother and baby post-delivery. It is very easy to get distracted by the need to care for a small newborn at the cost of missing a significant postpartum complication in the mother. Similarly, a distressed or ill mother may distract you from caring for the baby for long enough to allow the baby to become hypothermic.**

12.2 Abnormal presentations and lies

Definition

The relationship of the baby to the mother is important in labour. The following definitions help to describe them.

Lie – refers to the relationship of the long axis of the baby to that of the mother. These are **longitudinal**, **transverse** or **oblique** (Figure 12.1). If the lie changes it may be referred to as **unstable**.

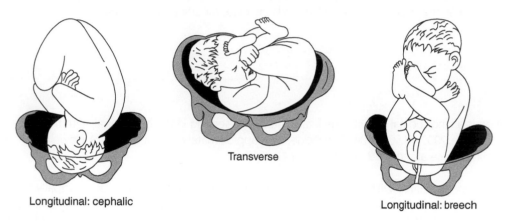

Longitudinal: cephalic

Transverse

Longitudinal: breech

Figure 12.1 Most common lies

Presentation – refers to the part of the baby that is presenting or foremost in the birth canal. The baby can present with its **head** (also known as cephalic presentation), **breech** (buttocks, feet or legs), **face**, **brow** or **shoulder** (Figure 12.2).

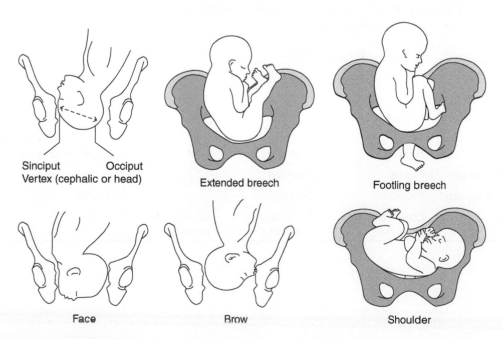

Sinciput   Occiput
Vertex (cephalic or head)

Extended breech

Footling breech

Face

Brow

Shoulder

Figure 12.2 Most common presentations

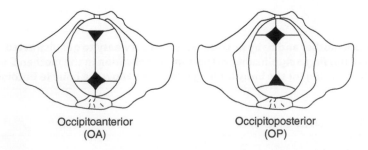

Occipitoanterior
(OA)

Occipitoposterior
(OP)

Figure 12.3 Most common positions

Position – refers to a reference point on the presenting part, and how it relates to the maternal pelvis. For example, the most common position is the **occipitoanterior** position (**OA** position). This occurs when the fetal occiput is directed towards the maternal symphysis or anteriorly (Figure 12.3). However, a common malposition is the **occipitoposterior** position (**OP** position). This occurs when the occiput is directed towards the maternal spine (ALSO, 2004).

12.3 Breech presentation

Definition

Breech presentation is a longitudinal lie with the fetal buttocks presenting in the birth canal, with the after-coming head in the uterine fundus (Boyle, 2002; ALSO, 2004). The incidence is approximately 20% at 28 weeks. However, as most babies turn spontaneously, the incidence at term is 3–4% (Impey et al., 2017a).

Breech presentations are associated with a higher perinatal mortality and morbidity rate, due principally to premature births, congenital malformations and birth asphyxia and trauma (Pritchard and MacDonald, 1980; Cheng and Hannah, 1993). The Term Breech Trial suggested that delivery by caesarean section is safer, with a lower newborn morbidity, for term pregnancies not yet in labour (Hannah, 2000). As first-line management, women diagnosed antenatally with a breech presentation at term should first be offered an external cephalic manipulation (an obstetric practitioner turning the fetus by hand) (Impey et al., 2017b).

Although the management of breech presentations has changed, there will still always be vaginal breech deliveries. These will occur as a result of undiagnosed breeches, rapid deliveries and patient choice. Therefore, all maternity care providers should be prepared for spontaneous breech deliveries.

Breech presentations can be classified as in Table 12.1.

Table 12.1 Classification of breech presentations

Type of breech presentation	Hips	Legs	Feet	Proportion of breech presentations
Frank (extended) breech	Flexed	Extended		65%
Complete (flexed) breech	Flexed	Flexed		25%
Footling breech	One or both extended	One or both extended	One or both presenting	10%

Risk factors

- Prematurity
- Previous breech presentation
- Low-lying placenta/placenta praevia
- Pelvic masses
- Bicornuate uterus
- Twins or higher multiples
- Polyhydramnios (too much liquor)
- Oligohydramnios (too little liquor)
- Fetal anomalies
- Grand multiparity

Diagnosis

The signs and symptoms will be similar to those of labour with a cephalic presentation. However, on inspection of the introitus, the following may be visible:

- The buttocks
- Feet or soles of the feet
- Swollen or bruised genitalia
- Meconium may be present (with the appearance of black toothpaste)

> **TOP TIP**
>
> **A breech may be confused with a bald-headed baby.**

> **TOP TIP**
>
> **Always check with the mother if she is aware of problems like an abnormal presentation.**

> **TOP TIP**
>
> **Always read the patient's hand-held notes. It may indicate within an alert box that this is a breech presentation.**

> **TOP TIP**
>
> **Assess to see if the birth is imminent, as this will influence your management.**

Pre-hospital management

1. Perform an obstetric primary survey following an ABCDEFG approach; address life-threatening findings in priority order.
2. Assess the signs of labour and determine which stage of labour the woman is in.
3. Get to the point quickly and attempt to identify potential complications, such as a preterm baby or cord prolapse.
4. If your assessment indicates that you can guarantee arriving at the hospital before delivery, commence transportation without delay.
5. Provide the receiving hospital with a pre-alert message.
6. However, if the birth seems imminent, or you have assessed that it will occur before you reach the hospital DO NOT commence transportation.
7. Request the urgent attendance of a community midwife.
8. If this is a preterm breech delivery, request a second ambulance, as per management of all preterm deliveries.
9. Prepare the area for a delivery; ensure neonatal resuscitation equipment is available, as well as Entonox® for the mother if required, warmed blankets (where possible) and delivery pack.
10. Support the woman in a semi-recumbent position, ensuring that her legs are supported in the lithotomy position (try using a couple of dining chairs to support the legs); alternatively the mother can support her own legs. Position her so that her buttocks are at the edge of either the bed or a sofa. Alternatively, the woman may choose to deliver on all fours, kneeling, standing or sitting on a birth stool.

11. The basic principle is not to interfere with spontaneous delivery of a breech baby, the golden rule being the 'hands off' approach.

12. The breech baby will rotate spontaneously to the sacroanterior position (back anterior to the mother). If this is not the case, then gentle rotation will be necessary to achieve this position. This will involve holding the fetal buttocks over the iliac crests, and gently rotating. DO NOT hold the legs or abdomen (Figure 12.4).

13. If the legs do not deliver spontaneously, they should be delivered by gentle flexion at the knee joint and abduction of the hip (Figure 12.5).

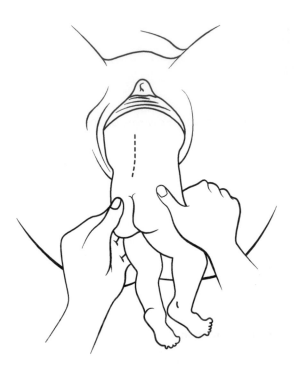

Figure 12.4 Manual rotation into the sacroanterior position

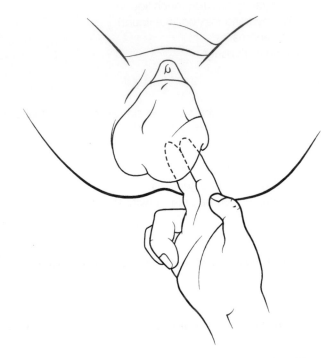

Figure 12.5 Flexion of the knee and abduction of the hip

14. DO NOT pull down a loop of cord.

15. If the arms do not deliver spontaneously, then assistance will be required using Løvset's manoeuvre (Figure 12.6). The baby should be lifted towards the maternal symphysis and rotated until one of the shoulders is in the anterior position.

16. Hold the baby by the pelvis – DO NOT hold the abdomen or legs.

17. A finger should be run over the shoulder and down to the elbow to deliver the arm across the front of the body.

18. Once the arm is delivered, the baby should then be gently rotated back to the sacroanterior position and if necessary the procedure repeated to deliver the other arm.

19. Once both arms have been delivered, ensure that the baby is rotated to the original position with the back anterior to the mother.

20. During delivery, wrap a towel or cover around the baby's body to ensure warmth, but DO NOT pull on the baby.

21. Once the nape of the neck is visible, it may be necessary to use the adapted Mauriceau–Smellie–Veit manoeuvre, designed to promote flexion of the head, in order to deliver it (Figure 12.7). This entails supporting the trunk of the baby over your arm so that it is in the horizontal position. With this supporting arm, place two fingers into the mother's vagina, and place them on the baby's cheekbones, one on each side. With the other hand, place your index finger and fourth finger and place on each of the baby's shoulders. Pressure should be placed on the occiput via the middle finger to ensure flexion of the head. Delivery of the head should then occur by flexion of the head. Always ensure that you explain to the mother what you are doing.

1.

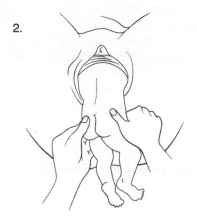

2.

3.

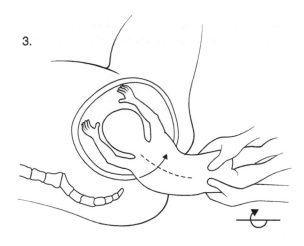

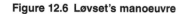

4.

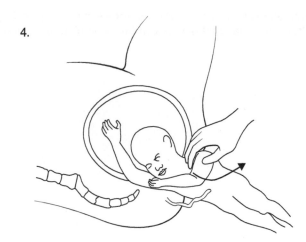

1. Here the arms are extended and cannot be delivered

2. The thumbs and fingers must grasp the baby's bony pelvis, **not** the abdomen

3. Gently flex the baby upwards ('sideways') Rotate baby 180° to bring the posterior arm to the front where it can be delivered now

4. Complete delivery of the arm Rotate the baby back 180° to deliver the second arm

Figure 12.6 Løvset's manoeuvre

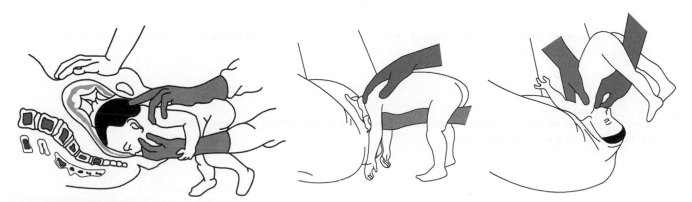

Figure 12.7 Adapted Mauriceau–Smellie–Veit manoeuvre

22. If the baby has still not delivered, place the mother in the McRobert's position (as for shoulder dystocia, see Section 12.10) and use suprapubic pressure to aid flexion and delivery of the head.

23. If the head still does not deliver and the midwife has not arrived, consider the most rapid way of obtaining skilled obstetric assistance through the appropriate channels, for example transferring the mother to the nearest maternity ward.

24. Once delivered, assess the baby in line with standard procedures. If neonatal resuscitation is required, follow the guidelines for newborn life support (see Chapter 14).

25. Manage the mother post-delivery as per guidelines for all vaginal deliveries, until the community midwife arrives.

TOP TIP

Remember the golden rule: 'hands off the breech' whenever possible.

TOP TIP

Pulling on the breech baby will complicate matters by leading to an extended head or nuchal arms, creating more difficulties and delay of the after-coming head (Figure 12.8). Incorrect handling of the baby may lead to internal organ damage.

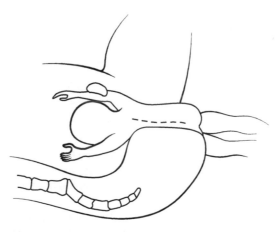

Figure 12.8 Extended head or nuchal arms

TOP TIP

When the mother chooses a semi-recumbent position for vaginal breech delivery, ensure the baby's back remains upwards during the delivery.

TOP TIP

When the mother chooses an 'all fours' position for vaginal breech delivery, ensure the front of the baby's abdomen remains upwards during the delivery.

TOP TIP

Do not delay. If you are unable to deliver the head immediately and no help has arrived, assess the most rapid way to obtain skilled obstetric assistance (Figure 12.9).

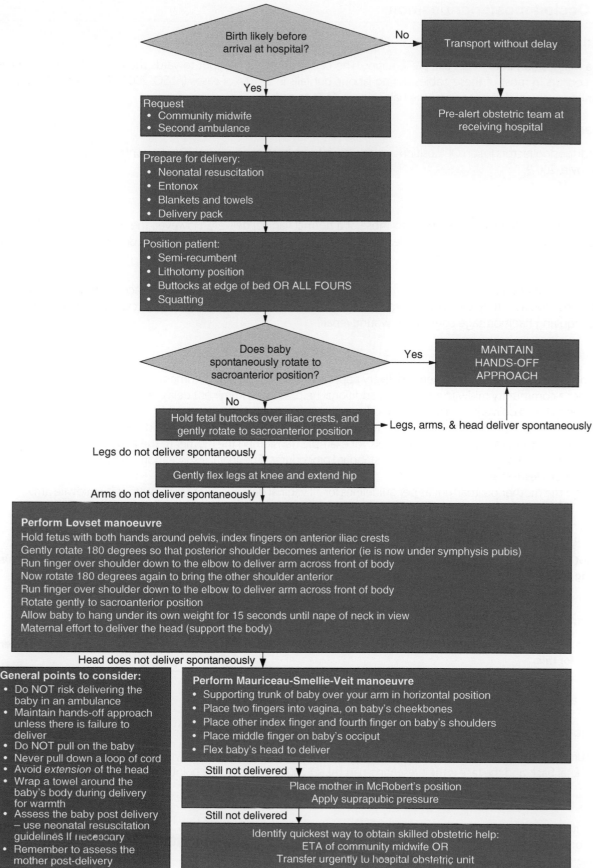

Figure 12.9 Algorithm for breech birth

12.4 Occipitoposterior position

Definition

This is a malposition in the cephalic presentation. The baby lies with its occiput towards the mother's spine. Spontaneous rotation occurs in most of these babies during labour, but fails in 5–10% of cases (ALSO, 2004). Therefore, in these cases, if spontaneous vaginal delivery occurs, the baby is born '**face to pubes**'.

Risk factors

The predisposing factors for an OP position are unknown, but it has been suggested that a contracted pelvis is a contributory factor (Boyle, 2002).

Diagnosis

The signs and symptoms may be similar to those of a normal vaginal delivery. However, the mother may feel like pushing prior to full dilatation of the cervix, so unless you can see anything visible at the introitus, do not always assume that the mother is in the second stage of labour.

The fetal head cannot deliver until the face has cleared the symphysis pubis. Therefore, this places strain on the perineum, and these babies look as if they will deliver through the rectum. Delivery of OP presentations can result in extensive perineal tearing, requiring haemorrhage control and wound repair.

Pre-hospital management

1. Manage as for all labouring women. If delivery appears imminent, DO NOT commence transportation.
2. Contact a community midwife and request additional help, as for all imminent deliveries.
3. Manage as for all deliveries, but be prepared for extensive perineal tearing.
4. If the head still does not deliver and the midwife has not arrived, consider the most rapid way of obtaining skilled obstetric assistance through the appropriate channels, for example transferring the mother to the nearest maternity ward.
5. Once delivered, assess the baby in line with standard procedures. If neonatal resuscitation is required, follow the guidelines for newborn resuscitation.
6. Manage the mother postpartum as per guidelines for all vaginal deliveries, until the community midwife arrives.

TOP TIP

Do not always assume that a woman is in the second stage of labour. The woman who has an OP baby may feel 'pushy' during the first stage of labour.

TOP TIP

A 'face to pubes' delivery may result in the mother sustaining extensive perineal lacerations, so care must be taken to assess for this.

12.5 Face presentation

Definition

This occurs in approximately one in 1000 deliveries (Gardberg et al., 2011). The head is hyperextended so the occiput is in contact with the fetal back, and the face is the presenting part (ALSO, 2004). The reference point of the baby is the mentum or chin.

Risk factors

- A large baby (fetal macrosomia)
- A contracted pelvis
- Enlargement of the neck caused by a cystic hygroma
- Multiple coils of cord around the neck
- OP position

Diagnosis

The signs and symptoms will be similar to those of a normal labour and presentation. However, parts of the face will be seen at the introitus and can be very misleading in appearance, as the face will be very oedematous and bruised. It can be confused with a breech presentation initially. Delivery of face presentations may result in extensive perineal tearing, requiring haemorrhage control and wound repair.

Pre-hospital management

1. Perform an obstetric primary survey following an ABCDEFG approach.
2. Manage as for all labouring women. If delivery is imminent, DO NOT commence transportation.
3. Contact a community midwife and request additional help, as for all imminent deliveries.
4. Manage as for all deliveries. The face of the baby will sweep the perineum, and the baby will deliver, but be prepared for an oedematous and very bruised baby. Warn the mother that this will be the case.
5. Be prepared to manage extensive perineal tearing.
6. Once delivered, assess the baby in line with standard procedures. If newborn resuscitation is required, follow the guidelines provided in Chapter 14. The baby born following a face presentation may have problems with its airway, due to oedema of the tongue.
7. Only mentoanterior face presentations will deliver vaginally (Figure 12.10). If you see a mentoposterior face presentation and the baby is more than 32 weeks' gestation, then you must consider transfer as such a baby is unlikely to deliver vaginally (Figure 12.11).
8. Manage the mother post-delivery as per guidelines, until the community midwife arrives.

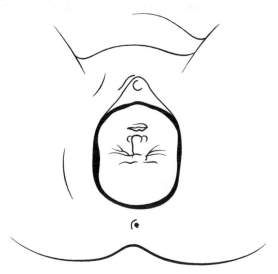

Figure 12.10 Mentoanterior face presentation

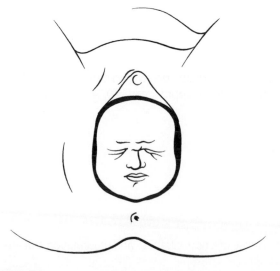

Figure 12.11 Mentoposterior face presentation

> **TOP TIP**
>
> 'Chin up – delivers; chin down – frown' (does not deliver).

> **TOP TIP**
>
> Take care not to initially confuse a face presentation with a breech presentation.

> **TOP TIP**
>
> The mother who delivers a baby with a face presentation may sustain extensive perineal lacerations, so care must be taken to assess for this.

12.6 Brow presentation

Definition

This is a rare presentation, approximately one in 5000 of all singleton deliveries (ALSO, 2004). The portion of the fetal head between the orbital ridge and the anterior fontanelle presents at the pelvic inlet. The causes of this are similar to those of a face presentation. It is possible for a brow presentation to convert to a face or vertex presentation.

Risk factors

- A large fetus (fetal macrosomia)
- A contracted pelvis
- Enlargement of the neck caused by a cystic hygroma
- Multiple coils of cord around the neck
- OP position

Diagnosis

Diagnosis is usually only by vaginal examination, and most brow presentations cannot deliver vaginally unless they are premature.

Pre-hospital management

Normal management is to move the obstetric patient to hospital as labour will not progress. A brow may convert to a face presentation or a vertex presentation.

12.7 Compound presentation

Definition

In this presentation, an extremity prolapses alongside the presenting part. This is usually a hand or a foot, but can on occasion be a hand and a foot. The incidence is thought to be approximately 0.04–0.14% of deliveries.

Risk factors

The causes are unknown, but it is more common in:

- Preterm infants
- Twins

Diagnosis

The signs and symptoms will be similar to those of a normal labour and presentation, but an extremity will be seen at the introitus.

Pre-hospital management

1. Perform an obstetric primary survey following an ABCDEFG approach.
2. Manage as for all other types of vaginal delivery.
3. The prolapsed limb may deliver spontaneously with the head, or the fetus may retract the prolapsed limb spontaneously. If you can access the limb, flick it gently and the baby may withdraw it.
4. Warn the mother of possible bruising to the limb.
5. If the prolapsed limb is delaying descent, assess to see whether the prolapsed limb may be gently elevated upward. If not, determine the most rapid way of obtaining skilled obstetric assistance.

12.8 Transverse and oblique lies

Definition

These occur when the long axis of the mother and fetus are approximately at right angles to each other. The fetus may lie in the transverse or oblique direction, with either the head or breech in the iliac fossa. The incidence is approximately one in 500 deliveries (Johanson et al., 2003). The presenting part is frequently the shoulder or cord. Transverse and oblique lies cannot deliver vaginally unless the lie is changed to longitudinal, and the uterus is at risk of rupture, with dire consequences for both mother and baby.

Risk factors

- Lax uterine muscles
- Placenta praevia
- Uterine anomalies
- Polyhydramnios
- Preterm fetus
- Twins and higher multiples
- Grand multiparity

Diagnosis

On abdominal palpation the uterus may feel broad, and no head or breech is found in the pelvis.

Pre-hospital management

1. Perform an obstetric primary survey following an ABCDEFG approach.
2. In the majority of cases delivery will not be imminent; therefore initiate transport without delay.
3. If the membranes rupture, assess for possible cord prolapse and manage appropriately.
4. If delivery appears imminent, which may be the case in extreme prematurity (babies less than 24 weeks) DO NOT initiate transportation. Ensure that a midwife has been contacted, and manage as per vaginal deliveries.

12.9 Multiple pregnancy

Definition

The incidence of spontaneous twin pregnancies in England and Wales during 2014 was 16 per 1000 births (ONS, 2014).

However, the rising use of infertility treatment increases not just the rate of twin pregnancies, but the incidence of triplets and quads. The incidence of perinatal mortality and morbidity is higher in multiple than singleton pregnancies. The main cause for this is the greater frequency of premature delivery and the associated complications (Boyle, 2002).

Maternal complications are common with multiple pregnancies, and these include pre-eclampsia, anaemia, placental abruption, placenta praevia and postpartum haemorrhage (Boyle, 2002; Cox and Grady, 2002).

Risk factors

- Fertility treatment
- Previous history of twins
- Familial history
- Multiparity

Diagnosis

Routine antenatal ultrasound scans will aid diagnosis of multiple pregnancies at an early gestation, and women will be closely monitored throughout their pregnancy. This will be documented within the patient's hand-held notes. However, if the woman has not received any antenatal care, the following may indicate an undiagnosed multiple pregnancy:

- The uterus may seem excessively large for the stage of pregnancy that the woman believes she is at (or she may deny that she is pregnant, or may actually not know)
- An excess of fetal parts may be palpable
- If the delivery of a baby has occurred and the uterus still seems large, suspect a second fetus. This may be more evident with the delivery of a small baby from a large uterus

> **TOP TIP**
>
> **Beware of the possibility of a multiple pregnancy in a woman who has received no antenatal care.**

Pre-hospital management

1. Perform an obstetric primary survey following an ABCDEFG approach; address life-threatening findings in priority order.
2. Assess to see whether the woman is in labour, and if so, determine which stage of labour she is in.
3. Get to the point quickly, and attempt to identify potential complications if the woman is in labour, such as:
    a. Dealing with the possible imminent delivery of two babies who may be preterm.
    b. Dealing with possible abnormal presentations of one or both babies.
    c. Cord prolapse.
    d. Postpartum haemorrhage.
4. Think about the other complications associated with multiple pregnancy, such as:
    a. Pre-eclampsia.
    b. Placental abruption.
    c. Anaemia.
5. If your assessment indicates that you can guarantee arriving at the hospital before delivery, commence transportation without delay.
6. Provide the receiving hospital with a pre-alert message.
7. However, if birth seems imminent, or you have assessed that it will occur before you reach the hospital **DO NOT** commence transportation. Instead:
    a. Request the attendance of a community midwife.
    b. Request a second ambulance as there will be three (or more) patients following delivery. **There is a high chance that the babies delivered will be preterm**.
8. Prepare the area for delivery. However, ensure that there are extra cord clamps, blankets and neonatal resuscitation equipment for two (or more) babies.
9. Support the woman in a comfortable position for delivery – usually semi-recumbent.
10. Manage the delivery as per usual guidance. Clamp and cut the first cord and await the descent of the second baby. **Do not wait long**. If there is no sign of descent of the second (or subsequent) baby, and the community midwife has not arrived, consider the most rapid way of obtaining skilled obstetric assistance, such as transferring the mother to the nearest maternity ward.
11. If the first and/or second twin is an abnormal presentation (e.g.breech), consider the most rapid way of obtaining skilled obstetric assistance, such as transferring the mother to the nearest maternity ward.
12. Once delivered, assess each baby in line with standard procedures. If newborn resuscitation is required, follow the guidelines in Chapter 14.
13. Manage the mother postpartum as per guidance for all vaginal deliveries, until the midwife arrives.

14. Be prepared for postpartum haemorrhage. Secure IV access as soon as possible.

15. Oxytocics should NOT be administered until the second (or final) baby has been delivered.

> **TOP TIP**
>
> **Do not wait long for the delivery of the second twin. Seek urgent obstetric assistance if the midwife has not arrived.**

12.10 Shoulder dystocia

Definition

Shoulder dystocia is described as a vaginal cephalic delivery requiring additional obstetric manoeuvres to deliver the fetus after the head has delivered and gentle traction has failed (Resnick, 1980). It manifests as an arrest of spontaneous delivery due to impaction of the anterior – or less commonly, the posterior – shoulder against the back of the symphysis pubis. The incidence is 0.58% and 0.70% of all deliveries (RCOG, 2014).

Risk factors

Antepartum

- Fetal macrosomia
- Maternal obesity
- Gestational diabetes
- Prolonged pregnancy
- Advanced maternal age
- Male fetus
- Excessive weight gain in pregnancy
- Previous shoulder dystocia
- Previous big baby

Intrapartum

- Prolonged first stage
- Prolonged second stage
- Assisted delivery

> **TOP TIP**
>
> **Remember that 50% of cases of shoulder dystocia do not have any risk factors and are associated with babies of normal birth weight (Gobbo et al., 2012).**

Diagnosis

In the late second stage you may notice 'head bobbing', where the head comes forward and is visible and then retracts between contractions. At delivery the 'turtle neck sign' may be seen, where the chin retracts tightly onto the perineum and the neck is not visible. The shoulders then fail to deliver with normal, **gentle** downward traction.

Pre-hospital management

It is important to remember the following principles:

- Do not pull, twist or bend the baby's neck
- Do not press on the uterine fundus
- Do not cut the cord before the baby is delivered

> **TOP TIP**
>
> **Never apply pressure to the fundus of the uterus – this will worsen impaction, may cause brachial plexus injury and rarely may result in uterine rupture.**

> **TOP TIP**
>
> **Excessive traction on the baby's neck risks significant damage to the brachial plexus.**

1. Perform an obstetric primary survey following an ABCDEFG approach.
2. Assess to see whether the woman is in labour, and, if so, determine which stage of labour she is in.
3. Get to the point quickly, identifying the potential problem.
4. Request the urgent attendance of a community midwife.
5. Attempt to deliver the anterior shoulder with gentle axial traction. ('Axial traction' means pulling gently in the line of the baby's neck and not pulling strongly downwards towards the floor, which can damage the brachial plexus.)
6. **If unsuccessful after two contractions, move on to McRobert's manoeuvre**. Around 90% of cases of shoulder dystocia will be managed successfully using this manoeuvre alone (in this position the pelvic diameters are increased and the angle of the pelvis is altered):
   a. The mother should be encouraged to move to the edge of the bed.
   b. The mother should be encouraged not to push, as this may increase impaction of the shoulder against the symphysis (RCOG, 2014).
   c. The mother should be asked to lie flat with only one pillow.
   d. The maternal hips should be flexed beyond 90°, causing the knees to be brought up towards the chest; the legs will abduct slightly because of the pregnant uterus.
   e. Now attempt to deliver the shoulders with gentle downwards traction (Figure 12.12a) with the contraction.

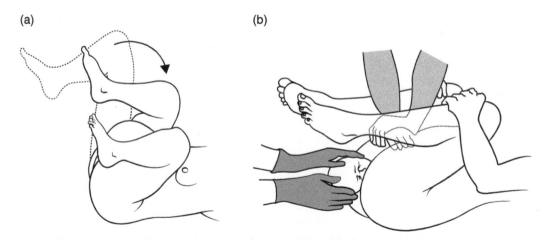

(a)   (b)

Figure 12.12 (a) McRobert's manoeuvre; (b) McRobert's with suprapubic pressure

7. **After two attempts, if the shoulders have not delivered, move on to suprapubic pressure**:
   a. Identify the side where the fetal back lies. This will be the opposite side to the direction the baby is facing.
   b. Ask whoever is helping to stand on the side of the baby's back (if the baby is facing left, stand on the mother's right, or vice versa).
   c. Ask your assistant to use their hands in CPR grip and place the heel of their hand two finger-breadths above the symphysis pubis behind the baby's shoulder.
   d. Ask the assistant to apply moderate pressure on the baby's shoulder pushing downwards and away from them *continuously* for no longer than 30 seconds. This will narrow the diameter of the shoulders and also push the anterior shoulder away from the midline, allowing it to pass under the symphysis pubis and deliver.
   e. The delivering practitioner should apply gentle traction downwards while suprapubic pressure is applied by the assistant (Figure 12.12b).
8. **After two attempts, if the shoulders have not delivered**:
   a. Ask your assistant to apply intermittent pressure on the shoulder by rocking gently backwards and forwards.
   b. The delivering practitioner should again try two further attempts to deliver while the assistant applies rocking suprapubic pressure.

9. **After two attempts, if the shoulders have not delivered:**
   a. Ask the mother to move into the 'all fours' position.
   b. Ensure that the mother's hips are well flexed, the bottom is elevated and her head is as low as possible (Figure 12.13).

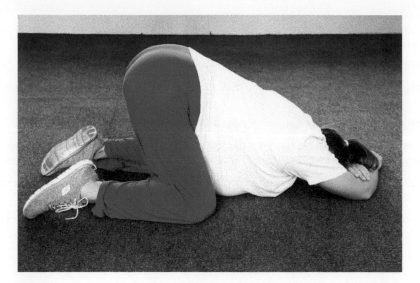

Figure 12.13 'All fours' position

   c. Attempt to deliver the baby in this position using gentle axial traction for up to 30 seconds (Figure 12.14).
   d. You will now be attempting to deliver the shoulder that is *uppermost*. Remember, this is *not* the shoulder that is stuck behind the symphysis pubis but once released, the baby will hopefully deliver.

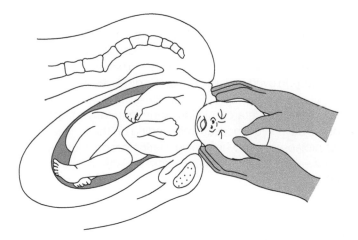

Figure 12.14 Delivery of the shoulder that is nearer the maternal back (mother in 'all fours' position)

10. **After two attempts, if the shoulders have not delivered transfer the patient without further delay to the nearest staffed obstetric unit.**
11. Move the mother into the ambulance and place in the 15–30° left lateral position.
12. If oxygen saturation on air falls below 94%, give oxygen.
13. Insert one or two large-bore cannulae en route (do NOT delay on scene to do this).
14. Provide the receiving hospital with a pre-alert message.

> **TOP TIP**
>
> **Suprapubic pressure should be applied from BEHIND the baby's anterior shoulder – look for the back of the head and apply pressure from the same side.**

HELPERR (Gobbo et al., 2012) is a mnemonic developed to guide management in shoulder dystocia. It starts with simple manoeuvres and moves on to encompass more complex manoeuvres which require *internal manipulation*. It is therefore suitable for use by *experienced* midwifery or obstetric staff.

The **HELLP-FOURS** mnemonic encompasses several of the initial manoeuvres and is more relevant for practitioners without obstetric/midwifery experience or expertise:

H – call for **H**elp: an early call to request a midwife (or obstetrician where relevant) to scene is the first and fundamental step

E – **E**dge of bed: positioning the patient at the edge of the bed will assist the practitioner greatly when applying appropriate axial traction

L – **L**ie the woman flat on the bed (use a pillow behind her head for comfort)

L – **L**egs: the McRobert's manoeuvre is simple and effective. Attempt to deliver the baby in this position by applying axial traction for up to 30 seconds. If delivery is not successful within 30 seconds, maintain the McRobert's position and add in the next manoeuvre ('P')

P – suprapubic **P**ressure: pressure applied either constantly or as in a 'CPR motion' may help the shoulder adduct or collapse anteriorly, and pass under the symphysis pubis

FOURS – roll the patient onto all FOURS: by moving to the 'all fours' position as in this position the pelvic diameter increases

---

TOP TIP

Use HELLP-FOURS as an aide-memoire when faced with shoulder dystocia.

12.11 Umbilical cord prolapse

Definition

Prolapsed cord is defined as descent of the umbilical cord below the presenting part in association with rupture of the membranes. If it lies adjacent to the presenting part, this is known as an occult prolapse; if it is below the presenting part, this is an overt prolapse. If the cord descends in front of the presenting part and before the membranes have ruptured, this is known as a cord presentation rather than prolapse. In overt prolapse the cord is displaced into the vagina and may be visible externally.

Prolapsed cord, of any type, can compromise the fetal circulation by intermittently compressing the cord between the mother and baby. This can cause fetal hypoxia, brain injury or death, depending on the degree and duration of the compression of the cord. Over 29% of cases of overt prolapsed cord where the gestation period is less than 37 weeks will result in a perinatal death, falling to 1% if gestation is 37 weeks or more. Fortunately, cord prolapse is a rare phenomenon, occurring in less than 0.25% of deliveries (Uygur et al., 2007).

Risk factors

- Prematurity (less than 34 weeks' gestation) and low birth weight
- Abnormal presentations; overt prolapse occurs in:
  - 0.5% cephalic and frank breech presentations
  - 5% complete breech presentations
  - 15% footling breech presentations
  - 20% transverse lie
- Occipitoposterior position
- Pelvic tumours
- Placenta praevia
- Cephalopelvic disproportion
- Polyhydramnios
- Multiparity
- Premature rupture of the membranes before the presenting part is engaged
- Long umbilical cord (Pritchard and MacDonald, 1980)

Diagnosis

Conducting a thorough patient assessment will reveal an overt cord prolapse at the introitus. Overt prolapse is most likely to be revealed at the point when the membranes rupture: always examine the vaginal opening once the waters have broken. However, obtaining an adequate obstetric history will also help to raise an index of suspicion for the risk of a prolapse occurring.

Occult prolapse is normally suspected on the basis of changes in the fetal heart rate, and is therefore likely to be difficult to identify with the limited monitoring available in the pre-hospital setting. Cord presentations can only be identified by palpation of the cord within the membranes. Making a diagnosis of cord presentation is rare in the pre-hospital setting without formal obstetric or midwifery training.

Pre-hospital management

Overt prolapsed cord is a time-critical emergency, requiring immediate transfer to the nearest obstetric unit.

1. Perform an obstetric primary survey following an ABCDEFG approach; address life-threatening findings in priority order.
2. Provided delivery is not imminent, the most urgent intervention is to elevate the presenting part of the fetus above the pelvic inlet to relieve compression of the cord:
   a. Positioning the patient with knees to chest (face to bed) with their buttocks raised is traditionally recommended for hospital use, but is impractical and unsafe in the pre-hospital setting and during transfer to the ambulance and transportation. Consequently, the mother should be placed in the 15–30° left lateral position with the hips raised by lowering the head of the ambulance trolley below the level of the pelvis (Figure 12.15) or raising the hips using blankets and other padding. Remember to use seatbelts to secure the patient during transfer and transportation.

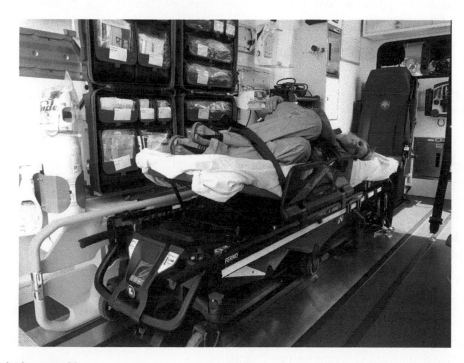

Figure 12.15 Trendelenburg position

   b. Apply manual pressure to the presenting part inside the vagina to lift it off the cord. Cradle the loop of cord gently in your palm to avoid pressing it against the vaginal wall and use the index and middle fingers to apply upward pressure to the presenting part. This pressure will need to be maintained until delivery in hospital (which is normally by caesarean section).
   c. As an alternative to manual pressure, a urinary catheter can be passed and the bladder filled with 500 ml of normal saline, after which the catheter is clamped until delivery. **Provided it can be achieved rapidly this should be done before moving the patient to the ambulance**.

3. Handling of the cord risks spasm and consequent fetal hypoxia. However, allowing the cord to become cold will also provoke spasm, and this is a significant risk in the pre-hospital setting. Consequently, if possible, small loops of cord should be replaced in the vagina. If the loops of cord are large and replacement in the vagina is not possible, they should be covered to avoid cooling with available dressings or sanitary pads.

4. Initiate transport to the nearest obstetric unit. Note that transfer of the patient to the ambulance can be challenging. Ideally, the trolley should be brought to the patient. If this is not practical, do NOT use a carry-chair, as this risks the mother sitting on the cord and increasing compression. If practical to do so and sufficient assistance is immediately available, the patient may be secured to a spine board in the 15–30° left lateral position with her hips raised on blankets. **This must NOT be allowed to delay initiation of transport** – if this is the case it is appropriate to bring the trolley as close to the patient as possible and ask her to walk to it.

5. Provide the receiving hospital with a pre-alert message.

> **TOP TIP**
>
> **Do NOT allow your preference for preventing the patient from walking to delay initiation of transport. Consider the effect on the prolapsed cord if transferring a patient on a carry-chair; always apply your own clinical judgement for the patient's best interests when deciding the safest and most expeditious method of getting to the ambulance.**

12.12 Umbilical cord rupture

Definition

Cord rupture is a tear in the umbilical cord. This can cause significant haemorrhage, hypovolaemic shock and even exsanguination of the fetus/newborn.

Risk factors

- Short cord
- Precipitous unassisted delivery (baby dangling by cord post-delivery)
- Premature babies (very friable cord)

Diagnosis

Tear in the cord – you may be alerted to this by the deteriorating condition of the newborn if the tear has occurred post-delivery between the cord clamp and the baby's abdomen, or by visible blood loss.

Pre-hospital management

This is a time-critical, life-threatening emergency: remember that even a small amount of blood loss from a newborn represents a significant proportion of their total circulating volume.

1. Apply direct pressure to the tear, preferably over a sterile swab.
2. If possible (that is, if the tear is not too close to the abdominal wall), position a clamp proximal to the tear.
3. Undertake an ABCDEFG neonatal primary survey and initiate newborn resuscitation based on the newborn's clinical condition.
4. Based on your assessment, consider a bolus of 10 ml/kg of normal saline (repeated as necessary). This can be delivered via IO needle, IV cannula or umbilical vein catheter (see Chapter 14).
5. Arrange immediate transport to the nearest hospital with appropriate facilities.
6. Provide the receiving hospital with a pre-alert message.

12.13 Other cord problems

Definition

A *short cord* is defined as an umbilical cord measuring less than 40 cm. However, a cord can be:

- *Absolutely* short – that is, its total length is limited
- *Relatively* short, as might be the case with an otherwise normal length cord being looped one or more times around the fetal neck

As the typical length of an umbilical cord is 55 cm or more, anything shorter may result in tension being placed on the cord. During labour, this can sometimes result in fetal asphyxia as the head descends. A short cord increases the risk that it will tear, resulting in life-threatening haemorrhage for the baby. Premature separation of the placenta, risking maternal haemorrhage and hypovolaemic shock for both mother and child, can also occur.

Diagnosis

An absolutely short cord will only be diagnosed after delivery. A relatively short cord (loops) will be seen at the time of delivery of the fetal head.

Pre-hospital management

Remember that this is potentially a life-threatening emergency for the mother and baby.

1. Deliver the baby normally as most will deliver through the loops of cord. If this is not the case, you may find it easier to position the baby with the head towards the perineum until you have unlooped the cord.
2. Avoid clamping and cutting the cord prior to delivery of the baby as, once cut, the circulation to the baby is stopped and therefore any delay in delivery could prove catastrophic.
3. Remember that premature placental separation may have occurred. You must therefore monitor the mother (using the ABCDEFG primary survey) for evidence of concealed or revealed bleeding and hypovolaemic shock. However, this is very rare.
4. If the cord is tearing or torn during or after delivery, immediately apply direct pressure to the tear and rapidly clamp and cut the cord, carefully ensuring that you clamp on both the mother's and baby's side of the cord proximal to the tear. This can be challenging if you cannot visualise the whole length of the cord during delivery, but failure to do so will result in catastrophic haemorrhage.
5. If the cord has torn, perform an ABCDEFG assessment of the newborn child. If there is evidence of significant haemorrhage or hypovolaemia, ensure bleeding at the tear is controlled by direct pressure and clamping of the cord and manage as for umbilical cord rupture.

TOP TIP

Avoid the temptation to routinely cut and clamp the cord if you note that it is looped around the neck. If delivery is delayed, the cord may be the baby's only supply of oxygenated blood and the baby will normally deliver through the loops.

Summary of key points

In preterm labour:

- Preterm labour is a significant predictor of neonatal morbidity and mortality
- Abnormal presentations and prolapsed cord are more common with preterm labour
- Preterm labour can proceed rapidly to delivery, so a careful assessment may prevent the need to deliver in the back of an ambulance
- Request the attendance of a midwife and second ambulance immediately you decide not to move a mother in preterm labour
- Hypothermia is a particular risk for a preterm newborn

In cord prolapse and other cord problems:

- Avoid the temptation to routinely cut and clamp the cord if you note that it is looped around the neck. If delivery is delayed, the cord may be the baby's only supply of oxygenated blood
- A torn umbilical cord can result in exsanguination of the fetus/newborn and must be managed immediately
- A patient with a prolapsed cord must be transported to an obstetrics unit without delay. DO NOT wait for additional resources to help you to move the patient

In malpresentations:

- A breech may be confused with a bald-headed baby
- Always check with the mother if she is aware of problems like an abnormal presentation
- Always read the patient's hand-held notes. It may indicate within an alert box that this is a breech presentation
- Assess to see if the birth is imminent, as this will influence your management
- Do not always assume that a woman is in the second stage of labour. The woman who has an OP baby may feel 'pushy' during the first stage of labour
- A 'face to pubes' delivery may result in the mother sustaining extensive perineal lacerations, so care must be taken to assess for this
- Take care not to initially confuse a face presentation with a breech presentation
- The mother who delivers a baby born through a face presentation may sustain extensive perineal lacerations, so care must be taken to assess for this

In multiple pregnancy:

- Oxytocics must not be given until the second/final baby has been delivered. If in doubt, do not administer
- Be prepared for preterm babies
- Be prepared for abnormal presentations and lies
- Do not wait long for the delivery of the second twin. Seek urgent obstetric assistance if the midwife has not arrived
- Be prepared for postpartum haemorrhage
- Beware of the possibility of a multiple pregnancy in a woman who has received no antenatal care

In shoulder dystocia:

- Remember that 50% of cases of shoulder dystocia do not have any risk factors and are associated with babies of normal birth weight
- Never apply pressure to the fundus of the uterus – this will worsen impaction, may cause brachial plexus injury and rarely may result in uterine rupture
- Use HELLP-FOURS as an aide-memoire when faced with shoulder dystocia

CHAPTER 13
Emergencies after delivery

Learning outcomes

After reading this chapter, you will be able to define, identify and describe the pre-hospital management of:
- Primary postpartum haemorrhage (PPH)
- Secondary PPH
- Trauma to the birth canal
- Acute uterine inversion
- Postpartum infection and puerperal sepsis
- Wound dehiscence

13.1 Primary postpartum haemorrhage

Definition

Primary PPH is defined as a blood loss of 500 ml or more within 24 hours of delivery and affects 3–5% of all deliveries. Massive PPH is clinically more important and may be life-threatening. A reasonable definition of massive PPH is 'loss of 50% of the blood volume within 3 hours of delivery'. Bleeding that is not so acute but continues at a rate of 150 ml/h or more, may also lead to unexpected maternal collapse. Bleeding that leads to haemodynamic instability would be another reasonable definition.

Between 2013 and 2015 there were 21 deaths that were reported as being related to haemorrhage, and this group continues to be the second leading cause of death occurring within 42 days of the end of pregnancy (MBRRACE-UK, 2017).

Risk factors

- Previous antepartum haemorrhage (APH) or PPH
- Long labour
- Anything that enlarges the uterus – multiple pregnancy, excess liquor (polyhydramnios), large baby
- Maternal age more than 40 years
- Obesity
- Multiparity (especially with five deliveries or more)
- Chorioamnionitis (intrauterine infection)
- Uterine fibroids (whether known or not)
- Partial separation of the placenta

The 'four Ts' is a simple tool to remind you of the common causes of primary PPH (RCOG, 2009a):

- Tone
- Trauma
- Tissue
- Thrombin

The most common cause (70%) is poor uterine tone. Trauma accounts for 20% and may involve any part of the genital tract and includes tears of the vulva, vagina or cervix, as well as uterine rupture, which should be considered in cases of labour with a uterine scar (most commonly a previous caesarean section). Tissue cases (10%) could involve retention of part of, or the whole, placenta. Thrombin refers to the development of disseminated intravascular coagulation (DIC), where blood clotting mechanisms are deranged and signs include bleeding from venous puncture sites; blood that is passed does not form clots.

Diagnosis

Blood loss is notoriously difficult to estimate accurately and there is a tendency to underestimate (for estimating blood loss, see Figure 6.2). Maternal physiological changes include a significant increase in circulating volume, which means that during pregnancy (and immediately after delivery), women do not exhibit overt warning signs of imminent collapse. In pregnancy, pulse and blood pressure are usually maintained in the normal range until blood loss exceeds 1000 ml. Tachycardia, tachypnoea and a slight recordable fall in systolic BP occur with blood loss of 1000–1500 ml. A systolic BP below 80 mmHg, associated with worsening tachycardia, tachypnoea and altered mental state, usually indicates a PPH in excess of 1500 ml.

If bleeding is more than expected it is recommended that early venous access is obtained with large-bore cannulae.

Although bleeding is obvious in most cases of major PPH, occasionally hypovolaemic shock can occur without overt bleeding. In these cases, consider haemorrhage that is 'concealed' – places where significant amounts of blood can accumulate include the paravaginal tissues (a haematoma of 2 litres or more may accumulate in the tissue space) and intra-abdominally (if there has been a uterine rupture).

> **TOP TIP**
>
> **In maternal haemorrhage, maternal collapse may not be preceded by warning signs such as rising pulse. Be prepared by gaining intravenous access en route to the hospital.**

> **TOP TIP**
>
> **Not all significant PPH is visible. In the presence of shock immediately post-delivery, consider 'hidden bleeding': paravaginal haematoma, rupture of a uterine scar (intra-abdominal bleeding) and broad ligament haematoma.**

Pre-hospital management

1. Fully assess ABCs – manage shock as described in Chapter 7.
2. Estimate the amount of visible bleeding (then 'double the estimate').
3. Consider the causes of primary PPH (the 'four Ts') – the commonest reason is uterine atony.
4. Feel for the uterine fundus – it normally feels 'hard and firm' and just reaches the umbilicus.
5. If the uterus feels 'soft and doughy', use the hand that is holding the fundus to 'rub up' a contraction (Box 13.1 and Figure 13.1).
6. Give a bolus dose of an oxytocic drug if bleeding continues (e.g. syntometrine IM or misoprostol PR).
7. With the mother's permission, check the vulval and perineal areas for obvious tears that might be bleeding. Local compression should be applied to control bleeding.
8. If possible, consider catheterisation to empty the bladder as this will help the uterus contract.
9. If the uterus is not contracting and haemorrhage is increasing, institute bimanual uterine compression (Box 13.2 and Figure 13.2). This will rarely be needed but may be a life-saving manoeuvre.
10. Arrange immediate transfer to a staffed obstetric unit.
11. Provide the receiving hospital with a pre-alert call.

12. The early administration of Tranexamic Acid (within 3 hours of delivery) has been shown to reduce mortality from PPH, following the initial administration of a uterotonic agent. The dosage of Tranexamic Acid is 1g IV, followed by a further dose if bleeding continues, or restarts after 30 minutes.

We consider it advisable to administer Tranexamic Acid, where indicated, to both pregnant and post-natal women.

Box 13.1 How to 'rub up' the uterus to encourage it to contract

1. Explain to the mother that this may be uncomfortable.
2. Firmly grasp with your hand the uterine fundus through the abdominal wall.
3. Gently 'massage' and 'squeeze' the uterus, which will encourage it to contract (Figure 13.1).
4. During this process, blood clots may be expelled and passed vaginally.
5. If this is effective, the bleeding will reduce and the uterus will become firm to touch and reduce in size.
6. You may need to continue this for several minutes.
7. If the uterus relaxes or bleeding continues, give an oxytocic drug.

Box 13.2 How to perform bimanual uterine compression

1. This is only required if haemorrhage becomes catastrophic. It will allow control of the bleeding during rapid transfer to hospital.
2. Explain to the mother that this will be very uncomfortable but is life-saving.
3. Use sterile gloves.
4. Insert two fingers into the vagina initially, then introduce the whole hand carefully and form a fist, with the back of your hand facing downwards.
5. Grasp the fundus of the uterus with the other hand and gently 'fold' the uterus forwards towards the pelvis.
6. Apply and maintain compression to the body of the uterus, between your two hands (Figure 13.2).

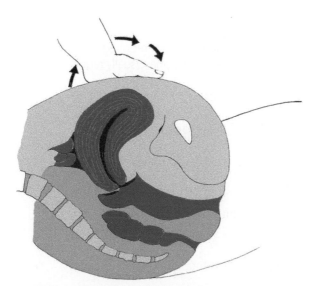

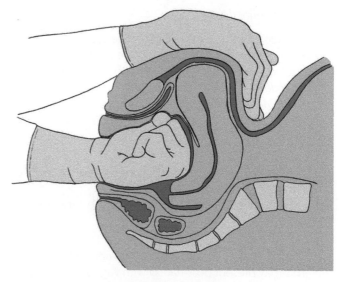

Figure 13.1 'Rubbing up' a uterine contraction: the left hand is cupped over the uterus and massages it with a firm, circular motion in a clockwise direction

Figure 13.2 Bimanual uterine compression

13.2 Secondary postpartum haemorrhage

Definition

This is bleeding that occurs between 24 hours and 6 weeks post-delivery. It most commonly occurs between the 5th and 10th day.

Risk factors

- Infection
- Retention of placental tissue

Diagnosis

- Bleeding following delivery may have temporarily ceased or reduced but then increases
- Bleeding can be severe
- Bleeding may be associated with cramps, generalised abdominal pain and back pain
- There may be an associated pyrexia and general malaise
- The blood loss may have an offensive odour

Pre-hospital management

1. Obtain a history of the delivery.
2. Treat as per shock guidelines (see Chapter 7).
3. Retain any tissue that has been passed and bring to the hospital.

TOP TIP

Estimation of blood loss is always very difficult. Assess the degree of loss then double the figure – you are less likely to underestimate blood loss using this method.

13.3 Trauma to the birth canal

Definition

Perineal trauma

This can be defined as:

- *First degree*, i.e. tear involving just the vaginal wall. If there is minimal bleeding, suturing is not required
- *Second degree*, i.e. tear involving the perineal muscles with a corresponding tear in the vagina. Usually requires suturing, but this may be done in the woman's home by the midwife
- *Third degree* includes the anal sphincter and always requires suturing in the hospital
- *Fourth degree* includes the anal mucosa and always requires suturing in the hospital
- Other lacerations: labial tears and grazes are common; if they are not bleeding, they do not require sutures

Cervical trauma

- The cervix may tear if the fetus passes through an incompletely dilated cervix
- It may be associated with other tears
- Occasionally, an obstetrician may cut the cervix in the case of head entrapment with a preterm breech delivery

Uterine trauma

- Usually associated with previous uterine surgery such as caesarean section or myomectomy
- This may present post-natally with vaginal bleeding and/or shock

Haematomas

Vulval – rupture of a vulval varix (varicose vein) or associated with perineal trauma. This can occur with a normal delivery and apparently intact perineum. An obvious painful swelling will be seen on one side of the vulva. It may present with severe buttock pain.

Vaginal – blood can accumulate in the space on either side of the vagina. There may or may not be pain and bleeding. This is a large potential space where several litres of blood may accumulate. Usually, nothing is visible on inspection of the vulva and the woman will eventually present with shock.

Broad ligament – the level of shock is out of proportion to the amount of blood loss seen.

> **TOP TIP**
>
> **The amount of concealed haemorrhage in the case of a haematoma is often significantly greater than the volume of blood seen – be prepared to manage severe shock.**

Risk factors

Trauma to the birth canal can happen with any delivery, but the following groups are at particular risk:

- Macrosomic baby
- Assisted delivery
- Shoulder dystocia

Diagnosis

- Can any tears be easily seen on the outside of the vulva?
- Is bleeding continuing despite a well-contracted uterus?
- Is there buttock pain?
- Consider whether there may be concealed haemorrhage

Pre-hospital management

1. Gain consent and inspect the woman's vulval area.
2. If the mother is shocked, institute care as for the standard management of shock and consider all causes.
3. If the mother is stable continue assessment of the vulva:
   a. Wearing gloves gently part the labia in order to complete your inspection.
   b. If there is a discrete bleeding point, apply local pressure with a pad, and if the bleeding is controlled await the arrival of the midwife.
   c. Rarely, direct pressure over a bleeding point or wound will be insufficient to control haemorrhage. Under these circumstances consider applying a pad containing a haemostatic agent to the wound. NB Haemostatic agents must NOT be used if the wound cannot be visualised.
   d. If a small non-bleeding tear is found, await the arrival of the midwife.

> **TOP TIP**
>
> **If the woman is shocked or has uncontrolled haemorrhage, treat as per PPH (see later) and initiate rapid transfer to hospital.**

> **TOP TIP**
>
> **Haemostatic agents must only be used in the event that continuous direct pressure to a visible wound fails to control bleeding.**

> **TOP TIP**
>
> **Haemostatic agents that produce an exothermic reaction should NOT be used.**

13.4 Acute uterine inversion

Definition

Inversion of the uterine fundus occurs in the immediate postpartum period. Inversion may be:

- **'Partial'** – where the inverted fundus remains within the body of the uterus
- **'Complete'** – where the inverted fundus protrudes through the cervix and in severe forms is visible outside the vagina

Only severe forms of inversion will be apparent in the pre-hospital setting. This is a rare complication affecting 1:2000 to 1:6400 deliveries. The commonest cause is traction on the cord without the other hand supporting the body of the uterus. Occasionally it can occur spontaneously, especially with excessive maternal pushing to try to deliver the placenta.

> **TOP TIP**
>
> **The use of cord traction by non-obstetric practitioners is not recommended as it risks uterine inversion.**

Risk factors

- Associated with a short umbilical cord
- Associated with uterine anomalies (e.g. uterine septum, 'double' uterus, congenital weakness – these are all rare)

Diagnosis

Early recognition is important to minimise maternal complications. Look for the following symptoms and signs:

- Severe lower abdominal pain during the third stage of labour (placental delivery)
- Firm, bulging mass at the vaginal entrance (placenta may or may not be attached)
- Uterus cannot be felt. Immediately post-delivery, the uterine fundus should be easily felt near the level of the umbilicus. In major inversion the uterus cannot be felt
- Shock that is disproportionate to the amount of visible bleeding (neurogenic shock)
- Shock associated with maternal bradycardia (this is due to excessive vagal stimulation because of 'traction' on the fallopian tubes and ovaries)

> **TOP TIP**
>
> **Consider uterine inversion in the presence of profound shock that is out of proportion to the amount of visible bleeding, particularly if there is a maternal bradycardia.**

Pre-hospital management

1. Institute active resuscitation in the presence of shock.
2. If oxygen saturation on air falls below 94%, give oxygen. If SpO_2 is less than 85% use a non-rebreathing mask; otherwise use a simple face mask. Aim for a target saturation of 94–98%.
3. If a bulging mass is visible at or outside the vaginal entrance, an immediate attempt should be made to replace the inverted uterus in the vagina. This simple manoeuvre may reverse the shock – see details in Box 13.3.
4. If bradycardia persists, gain intravenous access and administer atropine (500 micrograms to 3 mg maximum).
5. Prepare for rapid transfer to hospital.
6. En route to the hospital, obtain intravenous access.
7. Provide the hospital with a pre-alert call.
8. Ask for obstetric and midwifery staff to be informed of your estimated arrival time.

Box 13.3 Simple manoeuvres for immediate management of uterine inversion

1. Inform the patient that you are going to try to replace the womb inside the vagina and that this will be uncomfortable.
2. Ask the patient to lie on her back with her legs apart, so that you can easily reach the uterus.
3. Wear sterile gloves.
4. If the placenta is still attached DO NOT remove it.
5. Attempt to replace the uterus (and placenta if attached) back inside the vagina. Use a technique called 'taxis' (pronounced 'tax-iss'). Start by gently squeezing the part of the uterus nearest the vaginal entrance and gradually ease it back within the vagina. As the womb starts to go back inside, move your hands outwards and manipulate the rest of the uterus by gradually squeezing and pushing it inside.
6. Once the uterus is replaced in the vagina, the patient should remain lying flat. Avoid pressure on the abdomen to reduce the risk of the uterus coming back out.
7. If uterotonic medication such as Syntocinon® is available, this should be administered after uterine replacement.
8. Move the patient to an ambulance in as flat a position as possible, and maintain in this position during transfer to hospital.
9. If it is not possible to keep the patient flat after replacement of the uterus, it may be better to transfer to the ambulance first and attempt replacement there.
10. If it is not possible to replace the uterus or inversion recurs and is associated with shock and bradycardia, remember to administer atropine 500 microgram boluses titrated to effect.

Initial attempts to reposition the uterus in the pre-hospital situation

A single attempt at replacing the uterus within the vagina should be considered prior to transfer as this will reverse or prevent the development of shock (Box 13.3 and Figure 13.3).

In-hospital management

The obstetric management of acute uterine inversion in hospital initially involves the manoeuvres described above. If these are unsuccessful, the patient will be transferred to theatre and anaesthetised. The following options may be tried:

1. Attempt to reposition the uterus using taxis under general anaesthesia. Once the uterus is within the vagina, the obstetrician will try to reposition the uterus by forming a 'dimple' in the fundus and gradually pushing the womb 'outside in'.
2. If unsuccessful, 'hydrostatic' replacement is usually successful. This involves the obstetrician placing a hand in the vagina with a large-bore tube. The vaginal entrance is sealed with the other hand and several litres of sterile saline are introduced into the vagina. The vagina 'balloons' and the uterus gradually repositions itself.
3. Rarely, the abdomen will need to be opened to surgically to reposition the uterus from above.

(a)

(b)

(c)

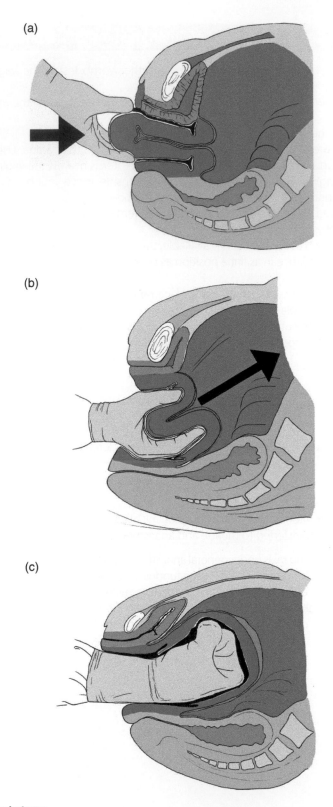

Figure 13.3 Replacing an inverted uterus

13.5 Postpartum infection and puerperal sepsis

Definition

This is an infection in the first 4–6 weeks after delivery that usually occurs in the upper genital tract. Ten per cent of women who have had a caesarean section will develop a postpartum infection, despite being given antibiotic prophylaxis at the time of surgery.

Sepsis is a life-threatening condition causing organ dysfunction that arises due to the body's response to infection. Sepsis is the primary cause of death from infection, especially if not recognised and treated promptly. Organ dysfunction may not be obvious and should be considered in any patient presenting with infection.

Of the women who died of causes directly related to pregnancy in 2013–15, 24 died from sepsis (MBRRACE-UK, 2017). Eight out of nine postpartum deaths from genital tract sepsis were due to group A *Streptococcus*. The rapid diagnosis and management of sepsis is critical to successful treatment.

The risk stratification tool (Table 13.1) published by NICE guides the practitioner to use the patient's history and physical examination results to grade the risk of severe illness or death from sepsis.

Table 13.1 Sepsis: recognition, diagnosis and early management for persons aged 12 years and over.

Category	High risk criteria	Moderate to high risk criteria	Low risk criteria
History	Objective evidence of new altered mental state	History from patient, friend or relative of new onset of altered behaviour or mental state History of acute deterioration of functional ability Impaired immune system (illness or drugs including oral steroids) Trauma, surgery or invasive procedures in the last 6 weeks	Normal behaviour
Respiratory	Raised respiratory rate: 25 breaths per minute or more New need for oxygen (40% FiO_2 or more) to maintain saturation more than 92% (or more than 88% in known chronic obstructive pulmonary disease)	Raised respiratory rate: 21–24 breaths per minute	No high risk or moderate to high risk criteria met
Blood pressure	Systolic blood pressure 90 mmHg or less or systolic blood pressure more than 40 mmHg below normal	Systolic blood pressure 91–100 mmHg	No high risk or moderate to high risk criteria met
Circulation and hydration	Raised heart rate: more than 130 beats per minute Not passed urine in previous 18 hours For catheterised patients, passed less than 0.5 ml/kg of urine per hour	Raised heart rate: 91–130 beats per minute (for pregnant women 100–130 beats per minute) or new onset arrhythmia Not passed urine in the past 12–18 hours For catheterised patients, passed 0.5–1 ml/kg of urine per hour	No high risk or moderate to high risk criteria met
Temperature		Tympanic temperature less than 36°C	
Skin	Mottled or ashen appearance Cyanosis of skin, lips or tongue Non-blanching rash of skin	Signs of potential infection, including redness, swelling or discharge at surgical site or breakdown of wound	No non-blanching rash

(Source: © NICE 2016 NG51 *Sepsis: recognition, diagnosis and early management*. Available from https://www.nice.org.uk/guidance/ng51. All rights reserved. Subject to Notice of rights. NICE guidance is prepared for the National Health Service in England. All NICE guidance is subject to regular review and may be updated or withdrawn. NICE accepts no responsibility for the use of its content in this product/publication)

Risk factors for puerperal sepsis

- Infections, which are more prevalent in pregnancy, such as urinary tract infection
- Impaired immune systems because of illness or drugs
- Invasive procedures such as caesarean section and instrumental deliveries
- Prolonged ruptured membranes before delivery
- Chorioamnionitis
- Prolonged labour
- Infected haematomas
- Retained swabs
- Gestational diabetes or diabetes

Diagnosis

Puerpural sepsis commonly presents as severe abdominal pain, high temperature and tenderness over the uterus, however it can be insidious in origin and progress rapidly to fulminating sepsis and death. Signs and symptoms can be vague and women with pelvic sepsis may present with diarrhoea, vomiting and abdominal pain – symptoms which are often attributed to gastroenteritis. Tachycardia, tachypnoea and altered mental state are early manifestations of sepsis, frequently preceded by fever and hypotension. Some patients with sepsis may not have a fever and may even by hypothermic.

The most common organisms identified in pregnant women dying from sepsis are Lancefield group A beta-haemolytic *Streptococcus* and *Escherichia coli*. Mixed infections with both Gram-positive and Gram-negative organisms are common, especially in chorioamnionitis. Coliform infection is particularly associated with urinary sepsis, preterm/premature rupture of membranes and cerclage. Anaerobes such as *Clostridium perfringens* (the cause of gas gangrene) are less commonly seen nowadays, with *Peptostreptococcus* and *Bacteroides* spp. predominating (RCOG, 2012).

Common sites of infection

Endometritis

- This is infection of the lining of the uterus
- It can happen after delivery or miscarriage
- It is more common after caesarean section or manual removal of the placenta
- It often presents with a temperature, lower abdominal pain and general malaise
- Lochia may be offensive and often heavy
- It may present as a PPH
- Sometimes the focus of infection will be some retained placental tissue
- Retained tissue may require removal under anaesthesia
- Rarely an abscess may develop

Urinary tract

- This is a very common type of infection
- It presents with urinary frequency and dysuria
- There may be loin pain which may signify pyelonephritis
- There are swinging temperature, sweats, fever and general malaise
- Nausea and vomiting may occur

Wound

- The wound becomes red, hot and inflamed
- There may be a hardened area above or below the wound where a haematoma or collection has formed
- The wound may open slightly allowing pus to drain out
- Pain can also be experienced at the wound site
- A temperature will be present (this may be swinging) and the woman may feel generally unwell

Perineal

A tear or episiotomy site can become infected. This often leads to:

- Wound break down
- Offensive lochia
- Temperature

Mastitis

- This is infection of the milk-producing gland tissue inside one or both breasts
- The breast may appear red and inflamed, and the mother will complain of pain in the affected breast
- Although uncomplicated mastitis may be treated at home with oral antibiotics, hospital admission is recommended for infections that are progressing rapidly or do not improve within 48 hours, or in women with signs of sepsis or who are immunocompromised
- The woman may need treatment with intravenous antibiotics, and if a breast abscess is suspected ultrasound assessment may be arranged. Breast abscesses are unlikely to resolve with antibiotic treatment alone and usually require surgical management with aspiration or incision and drainage
- The woman should be encouraged to continue breast feeding, or express milk if breast feeding has become too painful

Other infections

- Chest
- Viral, for example chicken pox and other childhood diseases

Pre-hospital management

This should be treated as per the shock guidelines given in Chapter 7.

This is a time-critical, life-threatening emergency requiring transport to hospital without unnecessary delay.

1. Perform an obstetric primary survey following an ABCDEFG approach; address life-threatening findings in priority order.
2. Consider the patient's position according to gestational stage and presenting condition.
3. Give oxygen if SpO_2 (on air) falls below 94%; aim for a target saturation of 94–98%.
4. Transport without delay to an appropriate emergency department, depending on local guidelines.
5. Provide the receiving hospital with a pre-alert message, ensuring that a senior on-call obstetrician is aware of your impending arrival if appropriate.
6. Insert a large-bore cannula en route (do NOT delay on scene to do this).
7. Administer crystalloids in 250 ml aliquots to maintain a systolic BP of >90 mmHg. Watch closely for further signs of circulatory decompensation.
8. Assess and document vital signs: respiratory rate, oxygen saturation, pulse rate (including quality), CRT and blood pressure, conscious level and temperature.
9. Point of care lactate testing, if available, may be done during transfer.
10. If appropriate intravenous broad-spectrum antibiotics are available before arrival at hospital, and transfer is likely to take more than 45 minutes, these can be administered before arrival. Ideally, blood for culture should be obtained before antibiotic administration, but this may not be possible prior to arrival at the hospital.
11. Take a detailed obstetric history (if patient's condition allows); request/review hand-held notes where possible.

13.6 Wound dehiscence

If a caesarean section wound has burst open: cover the wound with a moist, clean occlusive dressing and transport to hospital immediately.

Most other wounds should have a dry dressing applied. If the woman is systemically well and showing no signs of sepsis (see earlier) consider assessment and treatment in the pre-hospital setting rather than transporting to hospital.

Treatment of a localised would infection is with antibiotics, depending on the clinical condition, given orally or intravenously. If given orally the patient may be managed in the community with referral to the GP or midwife. Small areas of dehiscence rarely require resuturing.

Gas gangrene or necrotising fasciitis should be suspected if the wound looks necrotic, there are blisters on the skin surface or there is severe localised pain. If noted, transport to hospital for assessment.

TOP TIP

Check for a history of MRSA and alert the admitting hospital if there is a previous history of this.

Summary of key points

- The amount of concealed haemorrhage in the case of a haematoma is often significantly greater than the volume of blood seen – be prepared to manage severe shock
- If the woman is shocked or has uncontrolled haemorrhage, treat as per PPH and move rapidly to hospital (lights and sirens)
- In maternal haemorrhage, maternal collapse may not be preceded by warning signs such as a rising pulse. Be prepared by gaining intravenous access en route to hospital with two large-bore cannulae
- Not all significant PPH is visible. In the presence of shock immediately post-delivery, consider 'hidden bleeding': paravaginal haematoma or rupture of a uterine scar (intra-abdominal bleeding)
- The use of cord traction by non-obstetric practitioners is not recommended as it risks uterine inversion
- Consider uterine inversion in the presence of profound shock that is out of proportion to the amount of visible bleeding, particularly if there is a maternal bradycardia
- Estimation of blood loss is always very difficult. Assess the degree of loss then double the figure – you are less likely to underestimate blood loss using this method
- Women with sepsis may present with vague symptoms, and may not be pyrexial. They can become critically unwell rapidly
- In cases of postpartum infection check for a history of MRSA and alert the admitting hospital if there is a previous history
- In many cases of postpartum wound infection readmission to hospital is not necessary and simple infections can be dealt with by the midwife and GP

CHAPTER 14

Resuscitation of the baby at birth

Learning outcomes

After reading this chapter, you will be able to:
- Describe the normal physiology of a newborn
- Explain the difference between primary and terminal apnoea
- Describe and follow a strategy for the resuscitation of a newborn
- State how the response to resuscitation can be gauged

14.1 Introduction

The resuscitation of babies at birth is different from the resuscitation of all other age groups as it usually involves a process of assisted transition from intra- to extrauterine life, rather than recovery of a human with serious illness or injury. Knowledge of the physiology of normal transition and how interruption to transition, leading to hypoxia, affects this is essential to understand the process outlined in the algorithm (see Figure 14.7) for resuscitating newborn babies. The majority of babies will establish normal respiration and circulation without help. A tiny minority will not, and will require intervention. As some babies may be born unexpectedly out of hospital, in non-maternity settings within hospitals, or unwell as a result of peri-partum circumstances, it is important that clinicians working in 'receiving' specialties have an understanding of the differences between resuscitating an older child and a baby who has just been born. Ideally, someone trained in newborn resuscitation should be present at all deliveries. It is advisable that all those who attend deliveries regularly should have access to a course specifically concerned with newborn resuscitation.

14.2 Normal physiology

Successful transition at birth involves moving from a fetal state, where the lungs are fluid-filled and respiratory exchange occurs through the placenta, to that of a newly born baby whose air-filled lungs have successfully taken over that function. Preparation for this in a pregnancy progressing without incident is thought to begin in advance of labour, with detectable cellular changes occurring that may subsequently prime the lung tissues for reabsorption of the intra-alveolar fluid.

After delivery, a healthy term baby usually takes its first breath within 60–90 seconds. Stimuli for this first breath include exposure to the relative cold of the ex utero environment, the physical stimulus of being handled at delivery and hypoxia resulting from obstruction of the umbilical cord during clamping.

In a term baby, approximately 100 ml of fluid is cleared from the airways and alveoli, initially into the interstitial pulmonary tissue, and then later into the lymphatic and capillary systems.

Pre-Obstetric Emergency Training: A Practical Approach, Second Edition. Edited by Mark Woolcock.
© 2019 John Wiley & Sons Ltd. Published 2019 by John Wiley & Sons Ltd.

> **TOP TIP**
>
> **During vaginal delivery, only around 35 ml of fluid from the uppermost airways will be displaced by the physical forces experienced by the baby during passage through the birth canal.**

The respiratory pattern in newborn mammals has specifically evolved to efficiently replace the fluid in the airways and alveoli with air during the first few breaths. Animal studies show that at initiation of breathing, the inspiratory phase is longer than the expiratory phase (expiratory braking) and, in humans, expiration occurs against a partially closed glottis, creating backpressure (producing crying or sometimes a grunting sound). In a healthy baby the first spontaneous breaths may generate a negative inspiratory pressure of between −30 and −90 cmH$_2$O. This pressure is 10–15 times greater than that needed for later breathing but is necessary to overcome the viscosity of the fluid filling the airways, the surface tension of the fluid-filled lungs and the elastic recoil and resistance of the chest wall, lungs and airways. These powerful chest movements also aid displacement of fluid from the airways into the interstitial tissue before subsequent clearance into the lymphatics and ultimately the circulation. The combined effect of these events is to establish the baby's functional residual capacity (FRC).

Neonatal circulatory adaptation commences at the same time as the pulmonary changes. Lung inflation and alveolar distension releases vasomotor compounds that reduce the pulmonary vascular resistance as well as increasing oxygenation. Evidence shows that as pulmonary vascular resistance falls during establishment of the FRC, significant changes in stroke volume can be seen in the heart. Where the umbilical cord has been clamped prior to the first breath, a decrease in heart size is immediately seen, followed by return to its original size. This observation suggests a 'sink' effect, with blood being rapidly drawn into the pulmonary vessels as the lungs inflate with air during the first breaths, without access to placental blood to fill the emptied heart quickly and hence the observed decrease in size. The increase in size subsequently seen is likely due to the same large volume of blood returning to the left side of the heart from the expanded pulmonary circulation. Bradycardia has been noted in these babies consistent with the observed changes and, importantly, is not seen in babies who take their first breath before cord clamping. Circulatory adaptation proceeds with closure of the inter-atrial foramen, due to pressure changes as the pulmonary venous return to the left atrium increases, and finishes with functional, then permanent, closure of the ductus arteriosus over the following days.

14.3 Pathophysiology

When the placental oxygen supply is interrupted or severely reduced, the fetus will initiate respiratory movements (i.e. attempt to breathe) in response to hypoxia. If the interruption of oxygen from the placenta continues and these attempts at breathing fail to provide an alternative oxygen supply – as they will inevitably fail to do so in utero surrounded by amniotic fluid – the baby will become unconscious. If hypoxia continues, the higher respiratory centre becomes inactive and unable to continue to drive respiratory movements. The breathing therefore stops, usually within 2–3 minutes. This cessation of breathing is known as *primary* apnoea (Figure 14.1).

In the presence of hypoxia, a marked bradycardia will occur quickly. Intense peripheral vasoconstriction helps to maintain blood pressure with diversion of blood away from non-vital organs. The reduced heart rate allows a longer ventricular filling time, and thus an increased stroke volume, which also helps maintain blood pressure.

As hypoxia continues, primary apnoea is broken: loss of descending neural inhibition by the higher respiratory centre allows primitive spinal centres to initiate forceful, gasping breaths. These deep, irregular gasps are easily distinguishable from normal breaths as they only occur 6–12 times per minute and involve all the accessory muscles in a maximal, 'whole body' inspiratory effort. If this fails to draw air into the lungs and hypoxia continues, even this reflexive activity ceases and *terminal* apnoea begins. Without intervention, no further innate respiratory effort will occur. The time taken for such activity to cease is longer in the newly born baby than at any other time in life, taking up to 20 minutes.

The circulation is almost always maintained until *after* all respiratory activity ceases. This resilience is a feature of all newborn mammals at term and is largely due to the reserves of glycogen in the heart permitting prolonged, anaerobic generation of energy in the cardiomyocytes. Resuscitation is therefore relatively uncomplicated if undertaken before all respiratory activity has stopped. Once the lungs are aerated, oxygen will be carried to the heart and then to the brain provided the circulation is still functional (Figure 14.2). Recovery will then be rapid. *Most* babies who have *not* progressed to terminal apnoea will resuscitate themselves if their airway is open. Once gasping ceases, however, the circulation starts to fail and resuscitation becomes more difficult. Support for the circulation is then required in addition to support for the breathing (Figure 14.3).

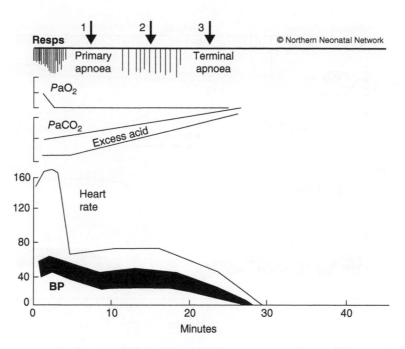

Figure 14.1 Response of a mammalian fetus to total, sustained asphyxia starting at time 0. (Reproduced with permission from the Northern Neonatal Network)

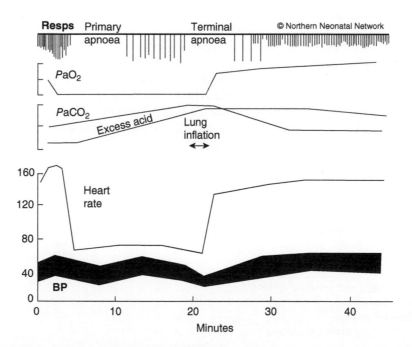

Figure 14.2 Effects of lung inflation and a brief period of ventilation for a baby born in early terminal apnoea but before failure of the circulation. (Reproduced with permission from the Northern Neonatal Network)

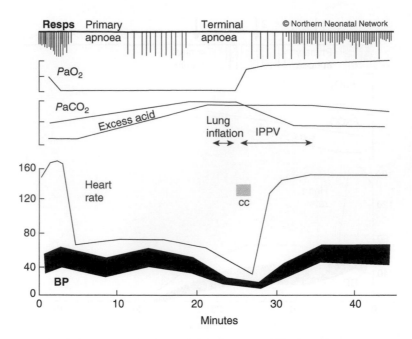

Figure 14.3 Response of a baby born in terminal apnoea. In this case lung inflation is not sufficient because the circulation is already failing. However, lung inflation delivers air to the lungs and then a brief period of chest compressions (CC) delivers oxygenated blood to the heart, which then responds. IPPV, intermittent positive pressure ventilation. (Reproduced with permission from the Northern Neonatal Network)

14.4 Equipment

For many newborn babies, especially those born outside the delivery suite, the need for resuscitation cannot be predicted. It is therefore useful to plan for such an eventuality. Equipment that may be required to resuscitate a newborn baby is listed in the following box. As a minimum, most babies can be resuscitated if there is access to: a firm, flat surface; warmth; a way to deliver air or oxygen to the lungs in a controlled fashion to displace the fluid present in the airways at delivery if the baby does not breath itself (ranging from using mouth-to-mouth to equipment-based techniques); and guidance from someone who is familiar with the process of newborn resuscitation (either as part of the resuscitation team or by telephone at the time of need). It is recognised that most ambulances and many settings which, although hospital based, have no access to obstetric services, will have limited access to equipment. The list provides a desired list, and not a minimum equipment inventory.

- A flat surface
- Radiant heat source and dry towels, or bubble wrap
- Plastic bag for term and preterm babies
- Suitable hats
- Suction with catheters of at least 12 Fr gauge
- Face masks
- Bag–valve–mask or T-piece with pressure-limiting device
- Source of oxygen and/or air
- Oropharyngeal (Guedel) airways
- Laryngoscopes with straight blades, size 0 and 1
- Nasogastric tubes
- Cord clamp
- Scissors
- Tracheal tubes sizes 2.5 to 4.0 mm
- Umbilical catheterisation equipment
- Adhesive tape
- Disposable gloves
- Saturation monitor/stethoscope

14.5 Strategy for assessing and resuscitating a baby at birth

Resuscitation is likely to be rapidly successful if commenced before the baby has progressed beyond the point at which its circulation has started to fail.

Babies in primary apnoea can usually resuscitate themselves if they have a clear airway. Unfortunately it is not possible, during the initial assessment, to reliably distinguish whether an apnoeic, newborn baby is in primary or terminal apnoea. A structured approach that will work in either situation must therefore be applied to *all* apnoeic babies. The structured approach is outlined here. In reality the first four steps (up to and including assessment) are completed simultaneously. After this, appropriate intervention can begin following an ABC approach:

- Call/shout for help
- Start the clock or note the time
- **Dry and wrap the baby in warmed dry towels**
- Maintain the baby's temperature
- **Assess the situation**:
  - Airway
  - Breathing
  - Chest compressions
  - (Drugs/vascular access)

Call for help

Ask for help if you expect or encounter any difficulty or if the delivery is outside the delivery suite.

Start the clock

Start the clock if available, or note the time of birth.

At birth

There is no need to rush to clamp the cord at delivery. It can be left unclamped while the following steps are completed:

- Dry the baby quickly and effectively
- Remove the wet towel and wrap in a fresh, dry, warm towel. (For very small or significantly preterm babies it is better to place the wet baby in a food-grade plastic bag – and later under a radiant heater)
- Put a hat on *all* babies regardless of gestation
- Assess the baby during and after drying and decide whether any intervention is going to be needed

If your assessment suggests that the baby is in need of resuscitation, clamp and cut the cord. If the baby appears well, wait for at least 1 minute from the complete delivery of the baby before clamping the cord.

If the baby is assessed as needing assistance/resuscitation then this becomes the priority. There is not yet sufficient evidence for advocating active resuscitation of the newborn human while still attached to the placenta by a functioning umbilical cord. Thus, the cord needs to be clamped and cut in order to deliver assistance/resuscitation.

Keep the baby warm

The normal temperature range for a newborn baby is 36.5–37.5 °C.

> **TOP TIP**
>
> **For each 1 °C decrease in admission temperature below this range in otherwise healthy, term, newborn babies, there is an associated increase in mortality of 28%.**

In environments likely to receive sick babies or infants, the room temperatures should be kept, as a baseline, as close as possible to the recommended minimum for term babies. Where delivery or admission of a newborn baby is imminent *outside* these environments, anticipation and active management of room temperature to achieve this baseline as quickly as possible is required: eliminate any draughts from the room (close windows and doors where possible) and heat the room to above 23 °C (term babies) or 25 °C (preterm babies).

Once delivered, dry the baby immediately and then wrap in a warm, dry towel. In addition to increased mortality risk, a cold baby has an increased rate of oxygen consumption and is more likely to become hypoglycaemic and acidotic. If this is not addressed at the beginning of resuscitation it is often forgotten. Most heat loss at delivery is caused by the baby being wet (evaporation) and in a draught (convection). Babies also have a large surface area-to-weight ratio exacerbating heat loss.

Ideally, an overhead heater or external heat source should be available and switched on, but drying effectively and wrapping the baby in a warm, dry towel with the head covered, preferably by a hat, is the most important factor in avoiding hypothermia. A naked, dry baby can still become hypothermic despite a warm room and a radiant heater, especially if there is a draught. In all babies, the head represents a significant part of the baby's surface area (see Section 14.9) so attention to providing a hat is invaluable in maintaining normothermia.

> **TOP TIP**
>
> **Some organisations advocate the use of bubble wrap to help maintain the temperature of a baby whilst out of hospital. This is often incorporated into the 'onion' wrapping technique where the first layer is a dry towel, the second layer is bubble wrap and the third layer is an aluminium foil blanket. This has proved to be highly effective, particularly in very cold regions.**

Out of hospital

Babies of all gestation ages born outside the normal delivery environment may benefit from placement in a food-grade polyethylene bag or wrap after drying and then swaddling. Alternatively, well newborn babies >30 weeks' gestation who are breathing may be dried and nursed with skin-to-skin contact (or kangaroo mother care) to maintain their temperature whilst they are transferred. Exposed skin should be covered to protect against cooling draughts.

Assessment of the newborn baby

During and immediately after drying and wrapping the baby, make a full ABC assessment.

A/B	• Breathing	Regular; gasp; none
C	• Heart rate	Fast; slow; very slow/absent
C	• Tone	Well flexed; reduced tone; floppy

Unlike resuscitation at other ages, *all* three items need to be assessed in parallel to be able to *then* decide on need for resuscitation and begin treatment and then assess its effect. This is different to the linear hierarchy of assessment and treatment used at other ages. In the newborn baby, *heart rate* and *breathing* provide the most useful information and are the *only* items that need regular reassessment during resuscitation to assess the effectiveness of intervention. At the initial assessment, however, taking note of the baby's tone can also be informative: a baby who is very floppy is likely to be unconscious, suggesting that the baby may have been subject to hypoxia.

Colour, while no longer formally assessed, is still a potentially useful indicator of status. Normal babies are born 'blue' and become 'pink' in the first minutes of life. A baby who is pale and white ('shut down' due to intense peripheral vasoconstriction) is more likely to be acidotic: this sort of appearance suggests significant cardiovascular response to peri-partum compromise.

Breathing movements and colour can be determined by observation during drying; tone can be evaluated at the same time. Heart rate is determined by auscultation of the heart using a stethoscope: this can be done during the drying by a second person *or* immediately afterwards if there is a lone responder.

Breathing

Most well term babies will take their first breath 60–90 seconds after delivery and will establish spontaneous, regular breathing sufficient to maintain a heart rate of ≥100 bpm within 3 minutes of birth. If there is no breathing (apnoea), gasping or irregular, ineffective breathing that persists after drying, intervention is required.

Heart rate

In the first couple of minutes, auscultating at the cardiac apex is the best method to assess the heart rate. Palpating peripheral pulses is not practical and is not recommended. Palpation of the umbilical pulse can only be relied upon if the palpable rate is ≥100 bpm. A rate less than this should be checked by auscultation as often it may not be possible to feel a cord pulse even though a heart rate is actually present.

If using a saturation monitor probe, it must be applied to the *right* (not left) hand or wrist in order to accurately reflect the pre-ductal saturations (which are most likely to reflect the oxygenation of blood returning to the left atrium – blood which is being distributed to the coronary arteries and cerebral circulation). A correctly applied pulse oximeter can give an accurate reading of heart rate and saturations within 90 seconds of application. Oxygen saturation levels in healthy babies in the first few minutes of life may be considerably lower than at other times. Attempting to judge oxygenation by assessing colour of the skin or mucous membranes is not reliable, but it is still worth noting the baby's colour at birth as well as whether, when and how it changes later in the resuscitation process. Very pale babies who remain pale and bradycardic after resuscitation may be hypovolaemic as well as acidotic. Similarly, tone immediately at birth should be assessed, and then changes noted as resuscitation progresses.

Time from birth	Acceptable pre-ductal SpO$_2$
2 min	60%
3 min	70%
4 min	80%
5 min	85%
10 min	90%

An accurate and prompt initial assessment of heart rate is vital because an increase in the heart rate will be the first sign of success during resuscitation.

Outcome of the initial assessment

Initial assessment will categorise the baby into one of the three following groups:

1. *Vigorous breathing or crying, good tone, heart rate ≥100 bpm.*
   These are healthy babies. They should be dried and kept warm but there is no need for immediate cord clamping. They can be given to their mothers and nursed skin-to-skin if this is appropriate and the baby can be protected from draughts by covering. The baby will remain warm through skin-to-skin contact under a cover and may also be put to the breast at this stage.

2. *Irregular or inadequate breathing or apnoea, normal or reduced tone, heart rate <100 bpm.*
   If gentle stimulation (drying will be an adequate stimulus in this situation) does not induce effective breathing, the cord will need to be clamped and cut to allow resuscitation to commence. After drying and wrapping has been completed, the airway should be opened. Most of these babies will improve with inflation of the lungs using a mask, and the heart rate should be used to assess the effect of this intervention. Some babies in this group will then require a period of ventilation by mask until they recover respiratory drive and are able to breathe for themselves.

3. *Breathing inadequately, gasping or apnoeic, globally floppy, heart rate very slow (<60 bpm)* **or** *absent and blue or pale.*
   Whether an apnoeic baby is in primary or terminal apnoea (Figure 14.1) the initial management is the same, though it will be quickly apparent that in this case delayed cord clamping is not appropriate. Cord milking ('stripping') has sometimes been advocated as an alternative to delayed cord clamping in babies who are in need of immediate assistance. However, the benefits of this have yet to be fully evaluated and thus it cannot be recommended except in the context of a properly conducted prospective study.

Dry and wrap the baby, assessing as you go and then commence resuscitation. Open the airway and then inflate the lungs. A reassessment of heart rate response then directs further resuscitation. In parallel, continued efficacy of mask ventilation should be monitored by watching for chest movement.

After assessment, resuscitation follows the broad categories of the structured approach seen in the algorithm (see Figure 14.7):

- Airway
- Breathing
- Circulation
- Drugs: may be useful in a few selected cases

Resuscitation of the newborn baby

Airway

To achieve an open airway, the baby should be positioned with the head in the neutral position (Figure 14.4). A newborn baby's head has a large, often moulded, occiput which tends to cause the neck to flex when the baby is supine on a flat surface. A 2 cm folded towel placed under the neck and shoulders may help to maintain the airway in a neutral position, and a jaw thrust may be needed to bring the tongue forward and open the airway, especially if the baby is floppy. However, overextension may also collapse the newborn baby's pharyngeal airway, leading to obstruction. If using a towel under the shoulders, care must be exercised to avoid such overextension of the neck.

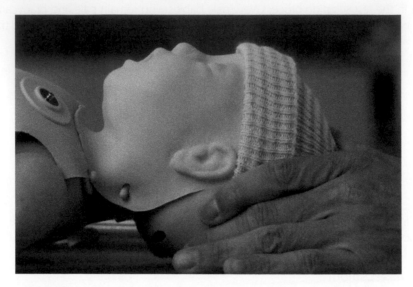

Figure 14.4 Neutral position in babies

Most secretions found in and around the oropharynx at birth are thin and rarely cause airway obstruction. Priority should be given in *all* babies to the application of a well-fitting mask and inflating the lungs once airway position and control is established. If, during resuscitation, there is concern that there might be an airway obstruction (e.g. if the heart rate is poor and the chest does not move with appropriately applied mask ventilation), the oropharynx can be directly visualised using a laryngoscope. Any obvious material obstructing the airway should be removed by gentle suction with a large-bore suction catheter. Deep pharyngeal suction without direct visualisation should not be performed as it may cause extensive soft tissue injury, vagal nerve-induced bradycardia and laryngospasm. Suction, if it is used, should not exceed −150 mmHg (−20.0 kPa).

Meconium aspiration

Meconium-stained liquor (light green tinge) is relatively common and occurs in up to 10% of births. Meconium *aspiration* is a *rare* event. Meconium aspiration usually happens in utero as the baby approaches term. It requires fetal compromise severe enough to cause both the reflexive passage of meconium *and* the onset of gasping respiratory movements. Because meconium has been inhaled before the delivery, it means that the previously widely advocated and used combined obstetric–neonatal strategy of suctioning the airways after delivery, has been shown to be of little use. Firstly, one large randomised trial has shown no advantage to suctioning the airway whilst the head is on the perineum. Secondly, another randomised trial has shown that routine intubation and suctioning of the baby's airway offers no advantage. Thirdly, a recent, small, randomised controlled trial has also demonstrated no difference in incidence of meconium aspiration syndrome in the most obtunded of babies who were subjected to tracheal intubation followed by suction and those who were not intubated. All that these procedures appear to do is delay the application of appropriate resuscitative measures to the baby in need. Thus when faced with a baby who has been born through meconium-stained liquor, and who needs assistance, initiation of resuscitative measures should be the priority *not* clearance of meconium.

From the perspective of effective resuscitation, the only type of meconium that may cause an immediate issue is that which is thick and viscid and which has the potential to block the airway. The presence of thick meconium should prompt *consideration* of direct visualisation of the oropharynx to remove any obstruction. However, again, the emphasis should be on initiating ventilation within the first minute of life in an apnoeic or ineffectively breathing baby. This should not be delayed and routine tracheal intubation is not recommended.

Breathing (aeration breaths and ventilation)

The first five breaths in term babies should be 'inflation' breaths in order to replace fluid in the alveoli with air. These should be 2–3-second sustained breaths ideally delivered using a continuous gas supply, a pressure-limited device (set at a limit of 30 cmH$_2$O) and an appropriately sized mask. Use a transparent, circular, soft mask big enough to cover the nose and mouth of the baby. If no such system is available then a 500 ml self-inflating bag and a blow-off valve set at 30–40 cmH$_2$O can be used (Figure 14.5). This is especially useful if compressed air or oxygen is not available. A smaller size of bag (<500 ml) will not have the capacity to sustain the inflation over 2–3 seconds and thus should not be used by choice unless no alternative exists. During these five breaths, it is important to remember that the chest may not be seen to move as fluid is displaced and replaced by air. After the five breaths, the first reassessment should be done.

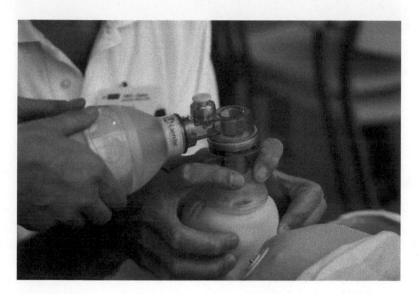

Figure 14.5 Airway opening in a newborn

Adequate ventilation is usually indicated by either a rapidly increasing heart rate or a heart rate that is maintained at ≥100 bpm. It is safe to assume the chest has been inflated successfully if the heart rate responds.

Once the chest is inflated and the heart rate has increased *or* the chest has been seen to move, then ventilation should be continued at a rate of 30–40 per minute using shorter breaths (no more than 1 second of inspiratory time). Continue ventilatory support until regular spontaneous breathing is established.

Where possible, start resuscitation of the newborn baby with air. There is now good evidence for its use in term babies and that oxygen toxicity causes significant morbidity in premature babies.

If the heart rate has not responded to the five inflation breaths then check that you have *seen* chest movement. Auscultation, by stethoscope, of fluid-filled lungs during the administration of inflation or ventilation breaths may erroneously detect 'breath' sounds *without* effective lung inflation. Go back and check airway opening manoeuvres and repeat the inflation breaths.

Circulation

If the heart rate remains very slow (<60 bpm) or absent, despite adequate lung inflation and subsequent ventilation for 30 seconds (with demonstrable chest movement), then chest compressions should be started.

Chest compressions in the newborn aim to move oxygenated blood from the lungs to the heart and coronary arteries; they are not intended to sustain cerebral circulation as they do in older children or adults. Once oxygenated blood reaches the coronary arteries it will usually result in a change from anaerobic energy generation to aerobic energy generation and, as a result, the heart rate will increase. This will then provide the required cardiac output to perfuse the vital organs. The blood you move using cardiac compressions *can only be oxygenated if the lungs have air in them*. Newborn cardiac compromise is almost always the result of respiratory failure and can only be effectively treated if effective ventilation is occurring.

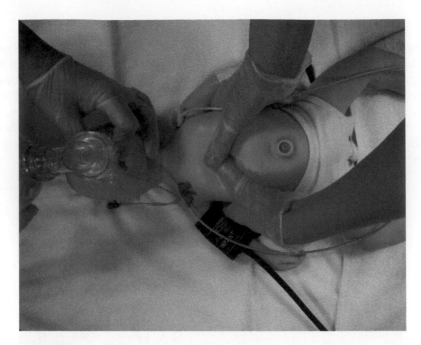

Figure 14.6 Hand-encircling technique

The most efficient way of delivering chest compressions in the newborn baby is to encircle the chest with both hands. The fingers lie behind the baby, supporting the back, and the thumbs are apposed over the lower third of the sternum (Figure 14.6). Overlapping the thumb tips is more effective than placing the thumb tips side by side, but is more likely to cause operator fatigue. Compress the chest briskly, *by one-third of the anteroposterior diameter* and ensure that *full recoil of the anterior chest wall is allowed* after each compression, before commencing the next compression. The relaxation phase is when the blood returns to the coronary arteries and therefore is essential to effective technique.

> **TOP TIP**
>
> **In newborn babies evidence clearly supports a synchronised ratio of three compressions for each ventilation breath (3:1 ratio) as the most effective ratio, aiming to achieve 120 events (90 compressions/30 ventilations) per minute.**

The purpose of chest compressions is to move *oxygenated* blood or drugs to the coronary arteries in order to initiate cardiac recovery. Thus there is no point in starting chest compressions before effective lung inflation has been established. Similarly, compressions are ineffective unless interposed by ventilation breaths of good quality. Therefore, the emphasis must be upon *good-quality breaths*, followed by effective compressions. Simultaneous delivery of compressions and breaths (otherwise known as chest compression with asynchronous ventilation, and used in older patients with a secure airway) should be avoided even when the baby is intubated. This is because compressions will reduce the effectiveness of any breath if the two coincide. It is usually only necessary to continue chest compressions for about 20–30 seconds before the heart responds with an increase in heart rate, thus reassessment of the heart rate at regular 30-second intervals is recommended. If chest compressions are *required* in resuscitation, the inspired concentration of oxygen should be increased if possible.

Once the heart rate is above 60 bpm and rising, chest compressions may be discontinued. Ventilation breaths will need to be continued, by whichever method has been used effectively thus far, until effective spontaneous breathing commences subsequently. In the absence of breathing starting spontaneously, formal mechanical ventilation may need to be instituted. The inspired oxygen concentration should be weaned guided by pulse oximetry.

Drugs

If adequate lung inflation and ventilation with effective cardiac compressions does not lead to the heart rate improving above 60 bpm, drugs should be considered. The most common reason for failure of the heart rate to respond is failure to achieve or maintain lung inflation, and there is *no point* in giving drugs unless the airway is open and the lungs have been inflated. Airway, breathing (i.e. observed chest movement) and chest compressions must be reassessed as adequate and effective before proceeding to drug therapy. Drugs are best administered via a centrally placed umbilical venous line, or if this is not possible an intraosseous needle is an alternative in term babies. The outcome is poor if drugs are *required* for resuscitation.

Adrenaline

The alpha-adrenergic effect of adrenaline increases coronary artery perfusion during resuscitation, enhancing oxygen delivery to the heart. In the presence of profound, unresponsive, bradycardia or circulatory standstill, 10 micrograms/kg (0.1 ml/kg of 1:10 000) of adrenaline may be given intravenously. This *must* be followed by a flush of 0.9% sodium chloride to ensure it reaches the circulation. Further doses of adrenaline 10–30 micrograms/kg (0.1–0.3 ml 1:10 000), again with a flush of 0.9% sodium chloride, may be tried if there is no response to the initial bolus. The tracheal route cannot be recommended, as there are insufficient data. However, if intratracheal instillation is tried, animal evidence suggests that doses of 50–100 micrograms/kg will be needed. These higher doses must *not* be given intravenously.

Bicarbonate

Any baby in terminal apnoea will have a significant metabolic component to the acidosis present. Acidosis depresses cardiac function. Sodium bicarbonate 1–2 mmol/kg (2–4 ml/kg of 4.2% solution) may be used to raise the pH and enhance the effects of oxygen and epinephrine in prolonged resuscitation, after adequate ventilation and circulation (with chest compressions) has been established. Bicarbonate use remains controversial and it should only be used in the absence of discernible cardiac output despite all resuscitative efforts, or in profound and unresponsive bradycardia. Its use is not recommended during short periods of cardiopulmonary resuscitation (CPR).

Glucose

Hypoglycaemia is associated with adverse neurological outcomes and worsened cerebral damage in neonatal animal models of asphyxia and resuscitation. Once the neonatal heart has consumed endogenous glycogen supplies, it also requires an exogenous energy source to continue functioning. Therefore, during prolonged resuscitation, it is appropriate to consider giving a slow bolus of 2.5 ml/kg of 10% glucose intravenously. Once a bolus has been given, provision of a secure intravenous dextrose infusion at a rate of 100 ml/kg/day of 10% glucose is needed to prevent rebound hypoglycaemia. Clinical evidence from paediatric patients suggests that hyperglycaemia after a hypoxic/ischaemic event is *not* harmful, whereas hypoglycaemia may well be. Many strip glucometers are not reliable in neonates and, wherever possible, should not be used for blood glucose estimation unless using the local laboratory arrangements incurs an excessive delay.

Fluid

Very occasionally hypovolaemia may be present because of known or suspected blood loss (antepartum haemorrhage, placenta/vasa praevia or bleeding from a separated but unclamped umbilical cord). Hypovolaemia secondary to loss of vascular tone following asphyxia is less common. Where a baby remains pale and shocked in appearance, or where there is a persistent bradycardia despite drug administration, intravascular volume expansion may be appropriate. A dose of 10 ml/kg of 0.9% sodium chloride (or other isotonic crystalloid) can be used safely. If blood *loss* is likely, especially where acute and severe, uncross-matched, cytomegalovirus negative, O rhesus (D) negative blood should be given in preference. Albumin (and other plasma substitutes) cannot be recommended. However, most newborn or neonatal resuscitations do not require administration of fluid unless there has been known blood loss or septicaemic shock.

As most newborn babies requiring resuscitation are not hypovolaemic, especially those born preterm, extreme caution should be exercised in order to avoid inappropriately excessive amounts of fluid boluses. Excessive intravascular volume expansion may cause worsened cardiac function in a heart subject to prolonged hypoxia, and is associated with increased rates of (cerebral) intraventricular haemorrhage and pulmonary haemorrhage in preterm babies.

Naloxone

This is not a drug of resuscitation to be given acutely. Occasionally, a baby *who has been effectively resuscitated* is pink and has a heart rate of ≥100 bpm, may not breathe spontaneously because of the possible effects of maternal opioid medications. If respiratory depressant effects are suspected the baby should be given naloxone IM (200 micrograms in a full-term baby). Smaller doses of 10 micrograms/kg will also reverse opioid sedation but the effect will only last a short time (20 minutes compared to a few hours after IM administration). Intravenous naloxone has a half-life shorter than the opiates it is meant to reverse, and there is no evidence to recommend intratracheal administration.

TOP TIP

Bicarbonate, glucose, fluid and naloxone should never be given intratracheally.

14.6 Response to resuscitation

The first indication of successful progress in resuscitation will be an increase in heart rate. Recovery of respiratory drive may be delayed. Babies in terminal apnoea will tend to gasp first as they recover before starting normal respirations (Figure 14.3). Those who were in primary apnoea are likely to start with normal breaths, which may commence at any stage of resuscitation. Depending on circulatory status, skin colour may recover quickly or slowly, but universally the tone (a proxy for consciousness) of the baby is the last key metric to improve once heart function, circulation and spontaneous, effective breathing are restored.

Discontinuation of resuscitation

The outcome for a baby with no detectable heart rate for more than 10 minutes after birth is likely to be very poor, with death or severe neurodisability the likeliest outcomes. Stopping resuscitation is a decision that should be made by the most senior clinicians present and ideally with input from those experienced in resuscitation of the newborn (which may mean consulting with neonatal teams, in other centres, by telephone or videoconferencing). This decision will depend on a range of variables including parental beliefs and expressed feelings about the potential for significant morbidity, likely aetiology for the presentation, potential reversibility of the cause, and availability of intensive care treatments including therapeutic hypothermia.

Where a heart rate has persisted at less than 60 bpm without improvement, during 10–15 minutes of continuous resuscitation, the decision to stop is much less clear. No evidence is available to recommend a universal approach beyond evaluation of the situation on a case-by-case basis by the resuscitating team and (ideally) senior clinicians.

A decision to stop resuscitation before 10 minutes, or not starting resuscitation at all, may be appropriate in situations of extreme prematurity (<23 weeks), birth weight of <400 g, or in the presence of lethal abnormalities such as anencephaly or confirmed trisomy 13 or 18. Such decisions should be taken by a senior member of the team, ideally a consultant in consultation with the parents and other team members.

Resuscitation is nearly always indicated in conditions with a high survival rate and acceptable morbidity.

14.7 Tracheal intubation

Most babies can be resuscitated using a mask system. Swedish data suggest that if this is applied effectively, only one in 500 babies actually *need* intubation. Tracheal intubation remains the gold standard in airway management *only* if the tracheal tube can be correctly placed, without interrupting ongoing ventilation, and without causing trauma to the oropharynx and trachea. It is especially useful in prolonged resuscitations, in managing extremely preterm babies and when a tracheal blockage is suspected. It should be considered if mask ventilation has failed, although the most common reason for this is poor positioning of the head with consequent failure to open the airway. It is, however, a common source of task fixation and can result in a significant interruption of resuscitation.

The technique of intubation is the same as for older infants. A usual-sized full-term newborn baby usually needs a 3.5 mm (internal diameter) tracheal tube, but 2.5, 3.0 and 4 mm tubes should also be available.

Tracheal tube placement must be assessed visually during intubation and in most cases will be confirmed by a rapid response in heart rate on ventilating via the endotracheal tube. An exhaled CO_2 detection system (either colorimetric or quantitative) is a rapid, and now widely available, adjunct to confirmation of correct tracheal tube placement in the presence of any cardiac output. Detection of exhaled CO_2 should be used to confirm tracheal tube placement but it should not be used in isolation; listening to air entry in both axillae may help avoid intubation of the right main bronchus which can give a 'false positive' capnographic test. A number of other false positive reactions can occur with direct contamination of the colorimetric detector by drugs used in the newborn setting.

14.8 Supraglottic airway device

A supraglottic airway (SGA) device may be considered as an alternative to a face mask for positive pressure ventilation among newborn babies weighing more than 2 kg or delivered ≥34 weeks' gestation. The use of a SGA device should be considered during resuscitation of the newborn baby if face mask ventilation is unsuccessful and tracheal intubation is unsuccessful or not feasible. There is limited evidence evaluating its use for newborn babies weighing <2 kg or delivered <34 weeks' gestation and none for babies who are receiving compressions.

Insertion of a SGA device should be undertaken only by those individuals who have been trained to use it.

14.9 Preterm babies

Unexpected deliveries outside delivery suites are more likely to be preterm. Moderately preterm babies (34–36 week's gestation) can be managed in the same way as term babies. Many babies born between 31 and 33 weeks' gestation, and *all* babies born before 31 weeks' gestation, need to be carefully supported during their transition to extrauterine life in order to prevent problems, rather than a need for resuscitation from a hypoxic event.

Premature babies are more likely to get cold (higher surface area to mass ratio), and more likely to become hypoglycaemic (fewer glycogen stores). There are now several trials that support keeping babies warm through the use of plastic bags placed over babies of <30 weeks' gestation (or <1000 g) without drying of unexposed body parts. Current European guidelines support wrapping the head and body (but not face) of all babies <32 weeks' gestation in polyethylene wrap or a bag where there is access to a radiant heater. The use of a radiant heater theoretically warms the wet baby through the plastic, trapping a warmed, humidified atmosphere around it to maintain thermal control (Box 14.1). In babies <32 weeks' gestation other interventions may also be needed to maintain temperature such as the use of a thermal mattress and warmed, humidified, respiratory gases when ventilated. Above 30 weeks' gestation, an alternative is to dry and wrap the baby in a dry warm towel in a similar fashion to babies born at term.

Box 14.1 Guidelines for the use of plastic bags for preterm babies (<32 weeks) at birth

1. Preterm babies born below 32 completed weeks' gestation may be placed in plastic bags or wrap for temperature stability during resuscitation. They should remain in the bag until they are on the neonatal intensive care unit (NICU) and the humidity within their incubator is at the desired level. This is a way of preventing evaporative heat loss and does not replace the use of incubators, etc. All efforts should still be made to maintain a high ambient temperature around babies born outside delivery suites.
2. At birth the baby should not be dried, but should be slipped straight into the prepared plastic bag or wrapping. There is no need to wrap the baby in a towel so long as this is done immediately after birth. This gives immediate humidity. The plastic bag only prevents evaporative heat loss – once in the bag, the baby should be placed under a radiant heater.
3. Suitable plastic bags are food-grade bags designed for microwaving and roasting. They should be large. The bag is prepared with a V cut in the closed end. Purpose-made bags and wraps are also available.
4. The bag should cover the baby from the shoulders to the feet, with the head protruding through the V cut. This is most easily performed if the hand is placed through the V, the head placed in the hand, and the bag drawn back down over the baby.
5. The head will stick out of the V cut and should be dried as usual and resuscitation commenced as per standard guidelines. If practical, a hat should be placed over the head to further reduce heat loss.
6. Standard resuscitation can be carried out without any limitations of access, but if the umbilicus is required for any access then a hole can be made above the area and the desired intervention done.
7. The bag should not be removed unless deemed necessary by the registrar or consultant.
8. After transfer to a neonatal unit and stabilising ventilation, if required, the baby's temperature should be recorded. The bag is only removed when the incubator humidity is satisfactory; further care is provided as per nursing protocols.
9. This is a potentially useful technique for keeping larger babies warm when born unexpectedly outside the delivery suite or in the community. However, it should be augmented by also wrapping with warm towels and ensuring a warm environment.

The more premature a baby, the less likely it is to establish adequate spontaneous respirations without assistance. Preterm babies of less than 32 weeks' gestation are likely to be deficient in surfactant, especially after unexpected or precipitate delivery. Surfactant, secreted by alveolar type II pneumocytes, reduces alveolar surface tension and prevents alveolar collapse on expiration. Small amounts of surfactant can be demonstrated from about 20 weeks' gestation, but a surge in production only occurs after 30–34 weeks. Surfactant is released at birth due to aeration and distension of the alveoli. Production is reduced by hypothermia (<35 °C), hypoxia and acidosis (pH <7.25). Surfactant deficiency can occur at any gestation but is especially likely in babies born before 30 weeks' gestation and many units will have a policy to address this issue based on the gestation at birth. Nasal continuous positive airways pressure (CPAP) is now widely used to stabilise preterm babies with respiratory distress and may avoid the need to intubate and ventilate many of these babies. If, however, intubation and ventilation is necessary, then exogenous surfactant should be given as soon as possible.

The lungs of preterm babies are more fragile than those of term babies and thus are much more susceptible to damage from overdistension. Therefore, it is appropriate to start with a lower inflation pressure of 20–25 cmH_2O but do not be afraid to increase this to 30 cmH_2O if there is no heart rate response. Using a positive end expiratory pressure (PEEP) helps prevent collapse of the airways during expiration and is normally given using a pressure of 5 cmH_2O. In most situations it will not be possible to measure the tidal volume of each breath given, and while seeing some chest movement helps confirm aeration of the lungs, very obvious chest wall movement in premature babies of less than 28 weeks' gestation may indicate excessive and potentially damaging tidal volumes. This should be avoided, therefore, especially in the context of a preterm baby with a heart rate ≥100 bpm and in whom there are adequate oxygen saturations.

Premature babies are more susceptible to the toxic effects of hyperoxia. Using a pulse oximeter to monitor both heart rate and oxygen saturation in these babies from birth makes stabilisation much easier. Exposing preterm babies at birth to high concentrations of oxygen can have significant long-term adverse effects. Ranges of pre-ductal oxygen saturation found in the first few minutes of life in well preterm babies are increasingly being reported, however normal values in well babies born before 32 weeks' gestation are based on small numbers. Trial data have shown clearly that starting resuscitation of the preterm baby in high (>65%) concentration inspired oxygen has no benefit over lower concentrations. The current guidance is that it is acceptable to start resuscitation of a preterm baby at an oxygen concentration between air and 30% as data do not exist currently to refine this range further. Additional oxygen should not be given if the oxygen saturations measured, at the right arm or wrist, are above the values given earlier in this chapter.

CPAP via mask versus intubation

As outlined in Section 14.7, tracheal intubation to 'secure' the airway is rarely needed in term babies. In addition, it carries with it the inherent risks of: delaying ongoing resuscitation due to task fixation; causing traumatic injury to oropharyngeal and tracheal tissue; and, at worst, irreversibly destabilising an otherwise well baby.

In preterm babies there is now good evidence from studies involving nearly 2500 babies under 30 weeks' gestation to suggest that effective initial respiratory support of spontaneously breathing babies with respiratory distress can be given using CPAP. Therefore, CPAP should be considered a first-line intervention for ongoing support in this population especially where personnel are not skilled in, or only infrequently practice, tracheal intubation. Where a mask plus T-piece system is being used for initial resuscitation, and a PEEP valve is available on the T-piece, CPAP may be given effectively by mask. Other dedicated CPAP devices utilising small nasal masks or prongs are available and are often found on paediatric high-dependency or level 1 neonatal ('special care') units.

Saturation monitoring

As outlined, pulse oximetry gives a quick and relatively accurate display of both heart rate and oxygen saturation that can be easily seen by all involved in the resuscitation. This is particularly useful when stabilising significantly preterm babies or when tempted to give additional oxygen to any baby. Once the oximeter is switched on, a reading can be obtained a few seconds faster if the probe is first attached to the right hand or wrist of the baby and only then connected to the machine. Once the heart rate is displayed with a good trace, it is likely that this will be more accurate than other commonly used methods of assessing heart rate.

Actions in the event of poor initial response to resuscitation

1. Check head position, airway and breathing.
2. Check for a technical fault:
   a. Is mask ventilation effective? Is there a significant leak around the mask? Observe chest movement.
   b. Is a longer inflation time or higher inflation pressure required?
   c. If the baby is intubated:
      i. Is the tracheal tube in the trachea? Auscultate both axillae, listen at the mouth for a large leak, and observe movement. Use an exhaled CO_2 detector to ensure tracheal tube position.
      ii. Is the tracheal tube in the right main bronchus? Auscultate both axillae and observe movement.
      iii. Is the tracheal tube blocked? Use an exhaled CO_2 detector to confirm tracheal position and patency of the tracheal tube. Remove it and re-try mask support if there is any concern that the tracheal tube is the problem.
   d. If starting in air then increase the oxygen concentration. This is least likely to be a cause of poor responsiveness, although if monitoring saturations it could be a cause for slow increase in observed saturations.

3. Does the baby have a pneumothorax? This occurs spontaneously in up to 1% of newborn babies, but pneumothoraces needing action in the maternity ward are exceptionally rare. Auscultate the chest for asymmetry of breath sounds. A cold light source can be used to transilluminate the chest – the pneumothorax may show as a hyper-illuminating area. If a tension pneumothorax is thought to be present clinically, a 21 G butterfly needle should be inserted through the second intercostal space in the mid-clavicular line. Alternatively, a 22 G cannula connected to a three-way tap may be used. Remember that you may well cause a pneumothorax during this procedure.

4. Does the baby remain cyanosed despite a regular breathing pattern, no increased work of breathing and with a good heart rate? There may be a congenital heart malformation, which may be duct dependent, or a persistent pulmonary hypertension.

5. If, after resuscitation, the baby is pink and has a good heart rate but is not breathing effectively, it may be suffering the effects of maternal opiates. Naloxone 200 micrograms may be given intramuscularly which should outlast the opiate effect.

6. Is there severe anaemia or hypovolaemia? In cases of large blood loss, 10–20 ml/kg O rhesus (D) negative blood should be given.

Birth outside the delivery suite

Whenever a baby is born unexpectedly, the greatest difficulty often lies in keeping it warm. Drying and wrapping, turning up the heating and closing windows and doors are all important in maintaining temperature. Special care must be taken to clamp and cut the cord to prevent blood loss.

Hospitals with an emergency medicine department should have guidelines for resuscitation at birth, summoning help and post-resuscitation transfer of babies born in, or admitted to, the department.

Babies born unexpectedly outside hospital are more likely to be preterm and at risk of rapidly becoming hypothermic. However, the principles of resuscitation are identical to the hospital setting. Transport will need to be discussed according to local guidelines. Remember the 'onion wrapping' technique described earlier in this chapter.

Communication with the parents

It is important that the team caring for the newborn baby informs the parents of the progress whenever possible. This is likely to be most difficult in unexpected deliveries so prior planning to cover the eventuality may be helpful. Decisions at the end of life must involve the parents whenever possible. All communication should be documented after the event.

Summary of key points

The approach to newborn resuscitation is summarised in the algorithm in Figure 14.7.

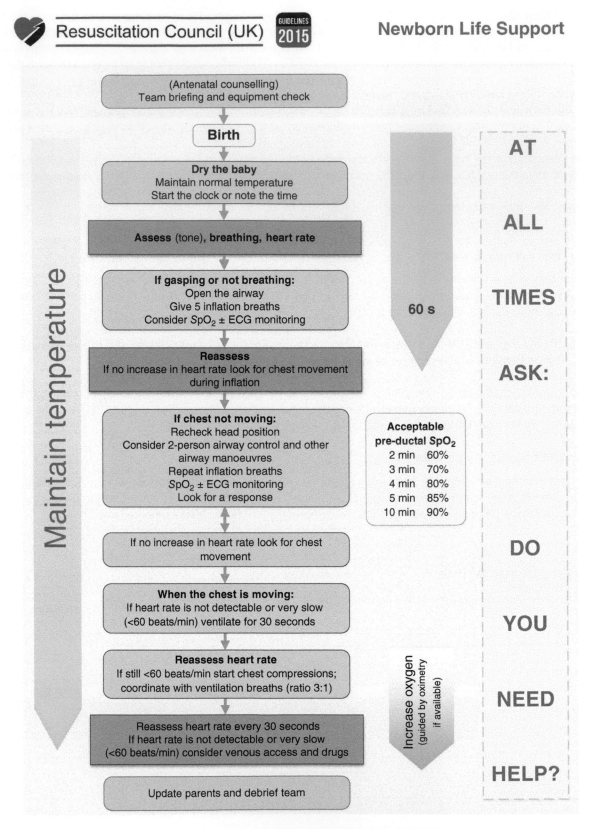

Figure 14.7 Newborn resuscitation algorithm. (Reproduced with kind permission of the Resuscitation Council (UK))

CHAPTER 15

Assessment and management of the post-gynaecological surgery patient

> **Learning outcomes**
>
> After reading this chapter, you will be able to:
> - Identify common types of gynaecological surgical procedures
> - Describe the pre-hospital management of complications following gynaecological surgery

Gynaecological surgical procedures may result in complications that present in a similar manner to emergencies in early pregnancy. Some of the more common procedures are described below. A thorough patient history will guide the practitioner in differentiating between complications in early pregnancy and complications post-surgery. Generally, the complications of gynaecological surgery are similar to those of any type of surgery.

15.1 Hysterectomy

Hysterectomy is performed for a variety of reasons including treatment of fibroids, endometriosis, chronic pelvic pain and cancer of the uterus, cervix or ovaries (NICE, 2007). The condition will dictate the type or extent of surgery required:

- *Total hysterectomy*: the uterus and cervix are removed (most common)
- *Subtotal hysterectomy*: the main body of the uterus is removed but the cervix is left in place
- *Total hysterectomy with bilateral salpingo-oophorectomy*: the uterus, cervix, fallopian tubes and ovaries are removed
- *Radical hysterectomy*: the uterus and surrounding tissues are removed including the fallopian tubes, part of the vagina, ovaries, lymph glands and omentum (NHS Choices, 2014)

There are three ways in which hysterectomy may be performed:

- *Abdominal hysterectomy*: this is performed through an incision made in the lower abdomen, usually horizontally above the pubic hair line, but may occasionally be via a vertical incision
- *Vaginal hysterectomy*: the uterus is removed via an incision made at the top of the vagina. This type of procedure generally allows for faster healing
- *Laparoscopic hysterectomy*: the uterus is removed through several small incisions in the abdomen. This is sometimes combined with a vaginal approach

Pre-Obstetric Emergency Training: A Practical Approach, Second Edition. Edited by Mark Woolcock.
© 2019 John Wiley & Sons Ltd. Published 2019 by John Wiley & Sons Ltd.

Recovery following laparoscopic and vaginal procedures is generally more rapid than following abdominal procedures. Patients will usually be fully mobile (although not fully recovered) within 1 week of laparoscopic and vaginal procedures. Full mobility often takes 2 weeks or more following an abdominal approach. It is normal to experience some bleeding, discharge and discomfort for several weeks following hysterectomy. However, bleeding near the vaginal vault may accumulate and may present with signs of infection and heavy, offensive bleeding or discharge.

Complications may occur with all types of hysterectomy. Early potential complications include trauma to blood vessels (haemorrhage requiring blood transfusion: 23:1000 women), bowel perforation (4:10 000 women) or bladder perforation (7:1000 women), which are more common with a laparoscopic approach (NICE, 2007; RCOG, 2009b). Frequent complications (which are more likely to be seen following discharge from hospital) include pelvic infection (2:1000 women), wound infection, urinary tract infection, wound haematoma and thromboembolic disorders (4:1000 women) (RCOG, 2009b).

15.2 Laparoscopy

Laparoscopy is performed as an investigative procedure, for example for pelvic pain or for treatment of gynaecological problems, including salpingectomy for ectopic pregnancy. It is important to be aware that, in some units, patients are discharged home the same day as surgery, even following hysterectomy, so it is vitally important not to assume that a patient discharged home the same day has only had minor surgery.

Carbon dioxide gas is introduced into the abdomen to allow better visibility via the laparoscope, which is passed into the abdomen usually via an incision at the umbilicus. This gas is slowly absorbed but can be uncomfortable post-surgery (NHS Choices, 2015b).

> **TOP TIP**
>
> **Patients often describe pain felt in the shoulder or shoulder blade region for 24–48 hours after laparoscopy. This is caused by stretching of the visceral peritoneal layer inside the abdomen.**

If blood vessel damage occurs, it is usually seen and corrected at the time of surgery. However, accidental damage to a loop of bowel may not be seen. Patients may be discharged home and present with increasing abdominal pain, infection or peritonitis any time from 1 to 5 days following laparoscopic surgery.

> **TOP TIP**
>
> **Bowel damage should always be suspected in patients presenting as unwell or with worsening abdominal pain in the days following laparoscopic surgery (see section on abdominal sepsis/peritonitis in Section 15.6).**

15.3 Large loop excision of transformation zone

Large loop excision of transformation zone (LLETZ) is carried out to remove abnormal cells identified at the opening of the cervix (often called 'pre-cancer'). It is either done alongside colposcopy or following colposcopy (examination of the cervix using a magnifying camera/scope). The cells are treated by drawing a wire across the site affected and passing an electrical current through the wire. It is common to have some bleeding for up to 4 weeks after the procedure while the site heals.

Cone biopsy may also be undertaken to remove abnormal cells, where a cone-shaped area of tissue is cut away from the cervix.

Women who have undergone any of these local treatments to the cervix may present with increasing bleeding or discharge which can be due to infection. Oral antibiotic treatment may suffice, but transport to hospital for assessment is required if bleeding is heavy and continuing, or if there are signs of sepsis.

15.4 Pelvic floor repair

This may be carried out to resolve a pelvic organ prolapse or to assist with symptoms of bladder incontinence.

Surgery is usually carried out vaginally, under general anaesthesia, but can be performed laparoscopically. Either route may involve suturing prolapsed vaginal tissue, plus or minus the insertion of a supporting mesh. Pelvic floor repair is commonly undertaken with a vaginal hysterectomy when the uterus itself is part of the prolapse.

It is normal to experience some bleeding, discharge and discomfort for several weeks after pelvic floor repair (with or without hysterectomy). Complications may include heavy, offensive bleeding or discharge, and the risk of venous thromboembolism or urinary tract infection (RCOG, 2015b).

15.5 Surgical uterine evacuation

This procedure is carried out for both miscarriage (SMOM or surgical management of miscarriage) and for terminating pregnancies (i.e. abortion). Complications include perforation or damage to the cervix (rare), secondary bleeding, the need for repeat procedure if not all products are removed (5:100 women) and pelvic infection (3:100 women) (RCOG, 2010).

15.6 Common complications of gynaecological surgery

Infection

Urinary tract

- This is a very common type of infection
- Patients present with:
  - Urinary frequency and dysuria
  - Loin pain (which may signify pyelonephritis)
  - Swinging temperature, sweats and fever
  - Feeling unwell
  - Nausea and vomiting may occur
- Treatment is usually with oral antibiotics that allow patients to be managed at home. However, if there are signs of sepsis hospital admission for IV antibiotics will be required

Wound infection

- The wound becomes painful, red, hot and inflamed
- There may be a hardened area above or below the wound where a haematoma has formed
- The wound may open slightly allowing pus to drain out
- Offensive smelling discharge may be present
- A temperature will be present (this may be swinging) and the woman may feel generally unwell
- Rarely the whole wound and the sheath itself will open producing a burst abdomen. Bowel may be seen through the opening:
  - Cover the wound with a moist, clean, occlusive dressing and transport to hospital immediately
- Most other wounds should have a dry dressing applied. Consider assessment and treatment in the pre-hospital setting rather than transporting to hospital unless the patient is systemically unwell
- Gas gangrene or necrotising fasciitis should be suspected if the wound looks necrotic or there are blisters on the skin surface, particularly if there is severe localised pain. Urgent transport to hospital, with a pre-alert call, is imperative
- Management includes thorough assessment of the wound and treatment varies depending on severity (local or systemic infection). If signs of systemic infection are present, referral to hospital is appropriate

Abdominal sepsis/peritonitis

Damage may occur to the bowel or other internal structures during surgery and may result in abdominal sepsis or peritonitis. Paralytic ileus, bowel perforation and intestinal obstruction may all occur postoperatively, and the differential diagnosis may be initially difficult. Paralytic ileus is common, and is usually self-limiting with supportive treatment in hospital. If bowel perforation occurs, and is not recognised at the time of surgery, it will present with signs of peritonitis, and urgent treatment is required. Intestinal obstruction may occur, possibly due to adhesions. In view of the difficulty of excluding a serious cause, all patients in this category require admission for assessment and management.

The signs/symptoms are:

- The patient will appear unwell
- Possible nausea and vomiting
- High temperature (which may progress to hypothermia in severe sepsis and septic shock)
- Tachycardia and possible hypotension in severe sepsis and septic shock
- Abdominal tenderness and distension, progressing to rebound guarding and rigidity

Management includes:

- ABC assessment
- Depending on severity of symptoms, obtain IV access en route
- Give IV fluids to maintain systolic blood pressure >90 mmHg
- Give high-flow oxygen
- Provide a pre-alert call to the nearest emergency department with surgical facilities
- In hospital, management includes IV antibiotics and possible surgical intervention (drainage of abscess or surgical lavage) (Rull, 2016)

Bleeding

Vaginal bleeding following hysterectomy may be due to release of a vault haematoma, or to fresh bleeding through the vagina and/or into the abdominal cavity from the surgical site. A vault haematoma is composed of old blood, and does not generally give cause for concern as there is no active bleeding. A high index of suspicion for intra-abdominal bleeding is crucial, as the diagnosis may be initially unclear, and urgent surgical intervention is required to control the bleeding.

Management includes:

- Assess severity according to haemorrhage criteria
- If the patient demonstrates signs of shock, administer oxygen to maintain oxygen saturations above 94%
- Insert a large-bore cannula and administer fluids as required to maintain systolic BP >90 mmHg
- Convey to hospital with a pre-alert call if indicated by signs and symptoms of shock or ongoing heavy bleeding

Deep vein thrombosis/pulmonary embolism

Patients who have undergone surgical procedures or hospitalisation are at increased risk for developing venous thromboembolism either peripherally (deep vein thrombosis (DVT), usually developing in the lower limbs) or centrally in the lungs (pulmonary embolism (PE)). There may be a history of calf pain or sudden collapse or sudden onset of difficulty in breathing.

Risk factors include:

- Extensive pelvic surgery
- Obesity
- Smoking
- Previous PE or DVT
- Immobilisation
- Previous treatment for malignancy in the past 6 months

Management includes:

- Assess and treat ABC, maintain airway and consider intubation if required
- Instigate cardiopulmonary resuscitation if there is no cardiac output
- Immediate transfer to nearest emergency department with pre-alert call
- Obtain IV access
- Thrombolysis in a post-surgical patient is a complex decision, which is unlikely to be advisable in the pre-hospital setting

---

Summary of key points

- Hysterectomy is performed for a variety of reasons, including treatment of fibroids, endometriosis, chronic pelvic pain and cancer of the uterus, cervix or ovaries
- There are three ways in which hysterectomy may be performed: abdominal hysterectomy, vaginal hysterectomy and laparoscopic hysterectomy
- Recovery following laparoscopic and vaginal procedures is generally more rapid than following abdominal procedures
- Frequent complications after discharge include pelvic infection, wound infection, urinary tract infection, wound haematoma and thromboembolic disorders
- Women who have undergone LLETZ may present with increasing bleeding or discharge which can be due to infection
- It is normal to experience some bleeding, discharge and discomfort for several weeks after pelvic floor repair (with or without hysterectomy)
- Common complications of gynaecological surgery include urinary tract infection, wound infection, abdominal sepsis and peritonitis, bleeding and venous thromboembolism

Abbreviations

The following obstetric abbreviations may be seen within the woman's hand-held notes and are used by both obstetricians and midwives. This list is not exhaustive. Full definitions can be found in the Glossary.

AFE	amniotic fluid embolism
AFLP	acute fatty liver of pregnancy
AFP	alpha fetoprotein
A/N	antenatal
APH	antepartum haemorrhage
BBA	born before arrival
Br	breech
Ceph	cephalic
CS	caesarean section
Cx	cervix
EDD	estimated date of delivery
EL	elective (referring to CS)
EM	emergency (referring to CS)
FHHR	fetal heart heard and regular
FMF	fetal movements felt
FMNF	fetal movements not felt
G	gravidity
IOL	induction of labour
IUD	intrauterine death
LMP	last menstrual period
LSCS	lower section caesarean section
MW	midwife
NND	neonatal death
Obs	obstetrics
P	parity
PHR	patient-held records
PN	postnatal
PPH	postpartum haemorrhage
Prem	premature/preterm
RPOC	retained products of conception
SROM	spontaneous rupture of membranes

Pre-Obstetric Emergency Training: A Practical Approach, Second Edition. Edited by Mark Woolcock.
© 2019 John Wiley & Sons Ltd. Published 2019 by John Wiley & Sons Ltd.

Glossary

The following obstetric terminology and abbreviations may be seen within the woman's hand-held notes, and are used by both obstetricians and midwives. Some hand-held notes list some of this terminology and its meaning in the front of the notes for the use of the woman and her partner. The following list is not exhaustive, but endeavours to cover the more commonly used terminology and abbreviations.

36 + 5: 36 weeks and 5 days pregnant.

5:10: 5 contractions in 10 minutes (= hyperstimulation).

Accoucher: French for a male obstetrician, a physician skilled in the art and science of managing pregnancy, labour and the puerperium (the time after delivery).

Active third stage: Delivery of the placenta using drugs and controlled cord traction to deliver the placenta.

Acute fatty liver of pregnancy (AFLP): Liver failure in late pregnancy, usually from unknown cause.

Alpha fetoprotein (AFP): One of the blood tests used to screen for Down's syndrome in the fetus.

Amniotic fluid embolism (AFE): Entry of liquor into the maternal circulation. A rare cause of maternal collapse.

Ampullary pregnancy: Ectopic pregnancy in the outer, wider part of the fallopian tube.

Antenatal (A/N) or antepartum: Events before birth.

Antepartum haemorrhage (APH): Bleeding from the birth canal before birth and after 24 weeks' gestation.

Apgar score: A system used to assess the condition of the baby during the first few minutes of birth.

APTT: Activated partial thromboplastin time.

Bicornuate uterus: Having two horns or horn-shaped branches. The uterus (normally unicornuate) can sometimes be bicornuate (with two branches, e.g. one at about 10:30 and the other at about 1:30).

Born before arrival (BBA): Unplanned delivery of the baby outside the hospital environment.

Breech (Br) presentation: Buttocks, legs or feet of the infant in the lower pole of the uterus.

Caesarean section (CS): Often referred to as **CS** or **LSCS** (lower segment caesarean section). EM = emergency, EL = elective.

Cephalic (Ceph): The fetal head. May also be known as the **vertex**.

Cervix (Cx): Lower portion of the neck of the uterus.

Pre-Obstetric Emergency Training: A Practical Approach, Second Edition. Edited by Mark Woolcock.
© 2019 John Wiley & Sons Ltd. Published 2019 by John Wiley & Sons Ltd.

Cord prolapse: When the membranes rupture and a cord is presenting in front of the baby.

CRP: C-reactive protein.

DIC: Disseminated intravascular coagulation.

Dystocia: Means 'difficult'. May be associated with shoulder dystocia or labour dystocia (protracted labour).

DVT: Deep venous thrombosis.

Early pregnancy: Pregnancies up to 24 weeks' gestation, especially before 20 weeks.

Early pregnancy assessment unit: Direct access for the management of women with early pregnancy problems.

Ectopic pregnancy: A pregnancy developing outside the uterus, usually in the fallopian tubes.

Engagement: Entry of the presenting part of the fetus (usually head) into the pelvis.

Episiotomy: A surgical incision made into the perineum to enlarge the vaginal orifice.

ESR: Erythrocyte sedimentation rate.

Estimated date of delivery (EDD): This is initially based on the **last menstrual period (LMP)**, then from a 12-week dating scan.

External cephalic version (ECV): Method of turning a baby from the breech position to head down position.

Fetal heart heard and regular (FHHR): Documented following auscultation of the fetal heart.

Fetal movements felt (FMF): Documented following enquiring about, or observing, fetal movements.

Fetal movements not felt (FMNF): Documented in the notes when a mother has not yet felt movements in early pregnancy or when movements cannot be felt in late pregnancy. This may be associated with fetal death.

Fetus: The unborn baby.

Gestation or gestational age: The completed weeks of pregnancy (not months). The mother's dates are usually calculated from the 12-week dating scan rather than the **last menstrual period (LMP)**. This will give a more accurate **expected date of delivery (EDD)**.

GFR: Glomerular filtration rate.

Gravid: Pregnant.

Gravidity (G): The number of times a woman has been pregnant, including the current pregnancy. This is regardless of the outcome of the pregnancies (for example it includes miscarriages). See also **parity**.

Haemolysis, elevated liver enzymes and low platelets (HELLP): A syndrome featuring a combination of 'H' for haemolysis (the breakdown of red blood cells), 'EL' for elevated liver enzymes and 'LP' for low platelet count (an essential blood clotting element).

Hb: Haemoglobin.

HELLP: Haemolysis, elevated liver enzymes and low platelet count.

Hyperstimulation: More than five contractions in 10 minutes.

Induction of labour (IOL): Labour that is artificially induced by various means.

Intrapartum: Events during labour.

Intrauterine: Within the uterus. For example, intrauterine transfer = transfer of a woman still pregnant.

Intrauterine death (IUD): Death of the fetus within the uterus.

Introitus: Entrance to the vagina.

Isthmus: Narrow middle portion of the fallopian tube.

Labour: Childbirth is described in three stages.

Last menstrual period (LMP): Used to work out initial estimated date of delivery.

Lie: The relationship between the long axis of the fetus to the uterus. This may be longitudinal, transverse or oblique.

Liquor: The fluid that fills the amniotic sac surrounding the baby.

Lithotomy: Position in which the patient is on their back with the hips and knees flexed and the thighs apart. The position is often used for vaginal examinations and childbirth.

Live birth: A baby born alive, irrespective of gestational age.

Lochia: The discharge from the uterus following childbirth, consisting of blood.

MCV: Mean corpuscular volume.

Meconium: Bright or dark green material which may be expelled from the fetal bowel whilst still *in utero*. It may be evident when the woman's waters have broken. It will be expelled from the baby following delivery.

Midwife (MW): A practitioner responsible for providing midwifery care to women during the antenatal, intrapartum and post-natal periods.

Miscarriage: The expulsion of the products of a pregnancy (in whole or part) before the end of the 24th week of pregnancy. It is associated with vaginal bleeding and pain.

Multigravida (or Multip): A pregnant woman who is not in her first pregnancy. A grand multip is a woman who has had a minimum of five births.

Multiple pregnancy: Pregnancy with more than one fetus.

Neonatal: The newborn baby.

Neonatal death (NND): Death of a live born baby within 28 days.

Obstetrics (Obs): A branch of medicine dealing with pregnancy, labour and the puerperium.

Occiput: The back of the fetal head.

Parity (P): Refers to the number of live births plus stillbirths a woman has had. For example, you may see **G3 P2** written. This means that this woman is in her third pregnancy, and has had two births. **G5 P2** means that the woman is in her fifth pregnancy but has only had two live births; the other two pregnancies may have been miscarriages. See also **gravidity**.

Pathway of care: This can be either high or low risk.

Patient-held records (PHR): Hand-held maternity notes that the woman carries with her throughout her pregnancy.

PE: Pulmonary embolism.

Perinatal: Around the time of birth.

Physiological second stage: Natural, without the use of drugs and controlled cord traction.

Placental location: Describes the relationship of the placenta in the uterus. It can be anterior, posterior, fundal, lateral or low. There are various ways of describing a low-lying placenta or praevia – distance from the internal cervical os (usually given in millimetres), partially covering the os or completely covering the os, or major or minor placenta praevia.

Position: Referring to the position of the baby in the uterus, using the fetal occiput as the denominator, for example occipitoanterior and occipitoposterior.

Postnatal (PN): After childbirth.

Postpartum: After labour.

Postpartum haemorrhage (PPH): Primary PPH means blood loss of more than 500 ml from the birth canal within 24 hours of delivery. Secondary PPH means excessive bleeding more than 24 hours after delivery.

Precipitate labour: A labour that is very fast. A precipitate delivery is therefore a rapid delivery.

Premature or preterm (Prem): Referring to labour or delivery before 37 completed weeks of gestation.

Presentation: The part of the baby that will be delivered first. For example, cephalic (head) or breech (buttocks).

Primigravida (Primip): A woman in her first pregnancy.

PT: Prothrombin time.

Puerperium: The 6-week period after the birth of the baby during which the mother's reproductive organs return to their pre-pregnant state.

Retained products of conception (RPOC): Products of conception refers to the combination of fetal and placental tissue.

Spontaneous rupture of membranes (SROM): When the 'waters break'.

Stillbirth (SB): A baby born after 24 weeks showing NO SIGNS OF LIFE at delivery. The fetus may have died days or even weeks before within the uterus. However, a baby of any gestation who shows signs of life has to be registered as a **live birth**. If you are involved with a pre-hospital birth in these circumstances, you must inform the relevant midwife and obstetrician.

Term: When pregnancy is completed within 37–42 weeks.

Trimester: A period of 3 months.

Tubal abortion: A term applied to an ectopic pregnancy when the conceptus is extruded from the fimbrial end of the fallopian tube.

Viability: The ability of the fetus to survive independently. Legally this is from 24 weeks' gestation.

WBC: Whole blood cell count.

References

ACOG (American College of Obstetricians and Gynecologists) (2012) Timing of umbilical cord clamping after birth. Committee Opinion No. 543. *Obstet Gynecol* 120: 1522–6.

ALSO (Advanced Life Support in Obstetrics) (2004) *Provider Manual*, 4th edn. Kansas: American Academy of Family Physicians.

Aslani A, Ng SC, Hurley M, McCarthy KF, McNicholas M, McCaul CL (2012) Accuracy of identification of the cricothyroid membrane in female subjects using palpation: an observational study. *Anesth Analg* 114: 987–92.

Battaloglu E, Porter K (2016) Management of pregnancy and obstetric complications in prehospital trauma care: faculty of prehospital care consensus guidelines. *Emerg Med J* 34(5): 318–25.

BECG (Birthplace in England Collaborative Group) (2011) Perinatal and maternal outcomes by planned place of birth for healthy women with low risk pregnancies: the Birthplace in England National Prospective Cohort Study. *BMJ* 343: d7400.

Bolam v. Friern Hospital Management Committee. 1, WLR 582; 1957.

Bose P, Regan F, Paterson-Brown S (2006) Improving the accuracy of estimated blood loss at obstetric haemorrhage using clinical reconstructions. *BJOG* 113(8): 919–24.

Boyle M (2002) *Emergencies Around Childbirth: A handbook for midwives*, 2nd edn. Buckingham: Open University Press.

Catchpole K (2010) Cited in Department of Health Human Factors Reference Group Interim Report, 1 March 2012, National Quality Board, March 2012. http://www.england.nhs.uk/ourwork/part-rel/nqb/ag-min/ (accessed March 2018).

CEMACH (Confidential Enquiry into Maternal and Child Health); Lewis G (ed.) (2007a) *Why Mothers Die 2003–2005. Report on confidential enquiries into maternal deaths in the United Kingdom*. London: CEMACH.

CEMACH (Confidential Enquiry into Maternal and Child Health); Lewis G (ed.) (2007b) *Saving Mothers' Lives: Reviewing maternal deaths to make motherhood safer: 2003–2005. The Seventh Report on Confidential Enquiries into Maternal Deaths in the United Kingdom*. London: CEMACH.

CEMACH (Confidential Enquiry into Maternal and Child Health) (2007c) *Diabetes in Pregnancy: Are we providing the best care? Findings of a national enquiry: England, Wales and Northern Ireland*. London: CEMACH.

CEMACH (Confidential Enquiry into Maternal and Child Health) (2007d) *Perinatal Mortality. 2005: England, Wales and Northern Ireland*. London: CEMACH.

Cheng M, Hannah M (1993) Breech delivery at term: a critical review of the literature. *Obstet Gynecol* 82: 605–18.

CMACE (Centre for Maternal and Child Enquiries); Lewis G (ed.) (2011) Saving Mothers' Lives: Reviewing maternal deaths to make motherhood safer: 2006–2008. The Eighth Report of the Confidential Enquiries into Maternal Deaths in the United Kingdom. *BJOG* 118 (Suppl 1): 1–203.

Cox C, Grady K (2002) *Managing Obstetric Emergencies*. Oxford: Bios Publishing.

Pre-Obstetric Emergency Training: A Practical Approach, Second Edition. Edited by Mark Woolcock.
© 2019 John Wiley & Sons Ltd. Published 2019 by John Wiley & Sons Ltd.

CPS (Crown Prosecution Service) (2009) *Policy for Prosecuting Cases of Rape*. London: CPS Communications Branch.

Dobbie AE, Cooke MW (2008) A descriptive review and discussion of litigation claims against ambulance services. *Emerg Med J* 25(7): 455–8.

DoH (Department of Health) (2001) *National Service Framework for Diabetes: Standards*. London: DoH.

DoH (Department of Health) (2007) *Maternity Matters: Choice, access and continuity of care in a safe service*. London: Crown Publishing. http://webarchive.nationalarchives.gov.uk/20130107105354/http:/www.dh.gov.uk/prod_consum_dh/groups/dh_digitalassets/@dh/@en/documents/digitalasset/dh_074199.pdf (accessed March 2018).

Duxbury F (2014) Domestic violence and abuse. In: Bewley S, Welch J (eds) *ABC of Domestic and Sexual Violence*. Chichester: John Wiley & Sons, pp. 9–16.

Elson CJ, Salim R, Potdar N, Chelty M, Ross JA, Kirk EJ on behalf of Royal College of Obstetricians and Gynaecologists (2016) Diagnosis and management of ectopic pregnancy. *BJOG* 123: e15–e55. http://onlinelibrary.wiley.com/doi/10.1111/1471-0528.14189/epdf (accessed March 2018).

ERC (European Resuscitation Council) (2015) *ERC Guidelines for 2015*. https://cprguidelines.eu (accessed March 2018).

Fellowes R, Woolcock M (eds) (2008) *Nancy Caroline's Emergency Care in the Streets*, 6th edn. Bridgwater: Jones & Bartlett.

Fortune P-M, Lawn C, Foëx B (2019) *Neonatal Adult and Paediatric Safe Transfer and Retrieval (NAPSTaR)*. Oxford: Wiley.

Gardberg M, Leonova Y, Laakkonen E (2011) Malpresentations – impact on mode of delivery. *Acta Obstet Gynecol Scand* 90(5): 540–2.

Gobbo R, Warren J, Hinshaw K (2012) *ALSO Syllabus Chapter I: Shoulder dystocia*. American Academy of Family Physicians.

Gorman N, Penna L (2015) Maternal collapse. *Obstet Gynaecol Reprod Med* 25: 5.

Hanna NJ, Black M, Sander JW, Smithson WH, Appleton R, Brown S, Fish DR (2002) *The National Sentinel Clinical Audit of Epilepsy-Related Death: Epilepsy – Death in the shadows*. London: The Stationery Office.

Hannah ME (2000) Planned caesarean section versus planned vaginal birth for breech presentation at term: randomised multicentre trial. *Lancet* 356: 1375–83.

HCPC (Health and Care Professions Council) (2012) *Confidentiality – Guidance for registrants*. London: HCPC.

HCPC (Health and Care Professions Council) (2016) *Standards of Conduct, Performance and Ethics*. London: HCPC.

Heslehurst N, Ells LJ, Batterham A, Wilkinson J, Summerbell CD (2007) Trends in maternal obesity incidence rates, demographic predictors and health inequalities in 36821 women over 15 years. *BJOG* 114: 187–94.

HTA (Human Tissue Authority) (2015) *Guidance on the Disposal of Pregnancy Remains Following Pregnancy Loss or Termination*. https://www.hta.gov.uk/sites/default/files/Guidance_on_the_disposal_of_pregnancy_remains.pdf (accessed March 2018).

Impey LWM, Murphy DJ, Griffiths M, Penna LK on behalf of the Royal College of Obstetricians and Gynaecologists (2017a) Management of breech presentation. *BJOG* 124(7): e151–77.

Impey LWM, Murphy DJ, Griffiths M, Penna LK on behalf of the Royal College of Obstetricians and Gynaecologists (2017b) External cephalic version and reducing the incidence of term breech presentation. *BJOG* doi 10.1111/1471-0528.14466.

Johanson J, Cox C, Grady K, Howell C (2003) *Managing Obstetric Emergencies and Trauma: The MOET course manual*. London: RCOG.

JRCALC (Joint Royal Colleges Ambulance Liaison Committee) (2016) *UK Ambulance Service Clinical Practice Guidelines 2016*. Bridgwater: Class Professional Publishing.

Knight M; UKOSS (UK Obstetric Surveillance System) (2007) Eclampsia in the United Kingdom 2005. *BJOG* 114(9): 1072–8.

Kohn LT, Corrigan J, Donaldson MS (2000) *To Err is Human: Building a safer health system*. Washington, DC: National Academy Press.

Leonard M, Bonacum D, Taggart B (2006) *Using SBAR to Improve Communication Between Caregivers*. London: Institute for Healthcare Improvement

Marshall J, Rayner M (eds) (2014) *Myles Textbook for Midwives*, 16th edn. Edinburgh: Churchill Livingstone Elsevier.

MBRRACE-UK; Knight M, Kenyon S, Brocklehurst P, Neilson J, Shakespeare J, Kurinczuk JJ (eds) on behalf of MBRRACE-UK (2014) *Saving Lives, Improving Mothers' Care – Lessons learned to inform future maternity care from the UK and Ireland Confidential Enquiries into Maternal Deaths and Morbidity 2009–12*. Oxford: National Perinatal Epidemiology Unit, University of Oxford.

MBRRACE-UK; Knight M, Tuffnell D, Kenyon S, Shakespeare J, Gray R, Kurinczuk JJ (eds) on behalf of MBRRACE-UK (2015a) *Saving Lives, Improving Mothers' Care – Surveillance of maternal deaths in the UK 2011–13 and lessons learned to inform maternity care from the UK and Ireland Confidential Enquiries into Maternal Deaths and Morbidity 2009–13.* Oxford: National Perinatal Epidemiology Unit, University of Oxford.

MBRRACE-UK; Manktelow BM, Smith LK, Evans TA, et al. on behalf of MBRRACE-UK (2015b) *Perinatal Mortality Surveillance Report UK. Perinatal deaths for births from January to December 2013.* Leicester: Infant Mortality and Morbidity Group, Department of Health Sciences, University of Leicester.

MBRRACE-UK; Knight M, Nair M, Tuffnell D, Kenyon S, Shakespeare J, Brocklehurst P, et al. on behalf of MBRRACE-UK (2016) *Saving Lives, Improving Mothers' Care – Surveillance of maternal deaths in the UK 2012–14 and lessons learned to inform maternity care from the UK and Ireland Confidential Enquiries into Maternal Deaths and Morbidity 2009–14.* Oxford: National Perinatal Epidemiology Unit, University of Oxford.

Murphy VE, Gibson P, Talbot PI, Clifton VL (2005) Severe asthma exacerbations during pregnancy. *Obstet Gynecol* 106: 1046–54.

Nathan HL, Duhig K, Hezelgrave NL, Chappell LC, Shennan AH (2015) Blood pressure measurement in pregnancy. *Obst Gynaecol* 17: 91–8.

NHS Choices (2014) *Hysterectomy.* http://www.nhs.uk/conditions/hysterectomy/Pages/Introduction.aspx (accessed March 2018).

NHS Choices (2015a) *Miscarriage – Causes.* http://www.nhs.uk/Conditions/Miscarriage/Pages/Causes.aspx (accessed March 2018).

NHS Choices (2015b) *Laparoscopy (Keyhole Surgery) – When it's used.* http://www.nhs.uk/Conditions/Laparoscopy/Pages/What-it-is-used-for.aspx (accessed March 2018).

NHS Digital (2017) *Statistics on Women's Smoking Status at Time of Delivery.* Leeds: Health and Social Care Information Centre, NHS Digital.

NHSLA (NHS Litigation Authority) (2012) *Ten Years of Maternity Claims: An analysis of NHS Litigation Authority data.* London: NHSLA.

NICE (National Institute for Health and Care Excellence) (2007) *Laparoscopic Techniques for Hysterectomy.* https://www.nice.org.uk/guidance/ipg239/resources/laparoscopic-techniques-for-hysterectomy-pdf-1899865344377797 (accessed March 2018).

NICE (National Institute for Health and Care Excellence) (2008) *Antenatal Care.* NICE Clinical Guideline 62. London: NICE.

NICE (National Institute for Health and Care Excellence) (2010) *Hypertension in Pregnancy: The management of hypertensive disorders during pregnancy.* NICE Clinical Guideline 107. London: NICE.

NICE (National Institute for Health and Care Excellence) (2012) *Ectopic Pregnancy and Miscarriage: Diagnosis and initial management in early pregnancy of ectopic pregnancy and miscarriage.* NICE Clinical Guideline 154. London: NICE.

NICE (National Institute for Health and Care Excellence) (2014) *Ectopic Pregnancy and Miscarriage.* NICE Quality Standard 69. London: NICE.

NICE (National Institute for Health and Care Excellence) (2016) *Sepsis: Recognition, diagnosis and early management.* NICE Guideline NG51. London: NICE.

NICE (National Institute for Health and Care Excellence) (2017) *Antenatal and Postnatal Mental Health: Clinical management and service guidance.* NICE Clinical Guideline 192. London: NICE (first published 2014, last updated 2017).

ONS (Office for National Statistics) (2014) *Birth Characteristics in England and Wales, 2014 – Statistical bulletin.* London: Office for National Statistics.

Pritchard JA, MacDonald PC (1980) Dystocia caused by abnormalities in presentation, position or development of the fetus. In: Pritchard JA, MacDonald (eds) *Williams Obstetrics.* Norwalk, CT: Appleton-Century-Crofts, pp. 787–96.

RCOG (Royal College of Obstetricians and Gynaecologists) (2001) *Thromboembolic Disease in Pregnancy and the Puerperium: Acute management.* Guideline No. 28. London: RCOG.

RCOG (Royal College of Obstetricians and Gynaecologists) (2009a) *Prevention and Management of Post Partum Haemorrhage.* Green-top Guideline No. 52. London RCOG.

RCOG (Royal College of Obstetricians and Gynaecologists) (2009b) *Abdominal Hysterectomy for Benign Conditions.* Consent Advice No. 4. LONDON: RCOG.

RCOG (Royal College of Obstetricians and Gynaecologists) (2010) *Surgical Evacuation of the Uterus for Early Pregnancy Loss.* Consent Advice No. 10. RCOG: London.

RCOG (Royal College of Obstetricians and Gynaecologists) (2011) *Maternal Collapse in Pregnancy and the Puerperium.* Green-top Guideline No. 56. London: RCOG.

RCOG (Royal College of Obstetricians and Gynaecologists) (2012) *Bacterial Sepsis in Pregnancy*. Green-top Guideline No. 64a. London: RCOG.

RCOG (Royal College of Obstetricians and Gynaecologists) (2014) *Shoulder Dystocia*. Green-top Guideline No. 42. London: RCOG.

RCOG (Royal College of Obstetricians and Gynaecologists) (2015a) *Obtaining Valid Consent*: Clinical Governance Advice No. 6. London: RCOG.

RCOG (Royal College of Obstetricians and Gynaecologists) (2015b) *Recovering Well – Information for you after a Pelvic Floor Repair Operation*. London: RCOG.

RCUK (Resuscitation Council (UK)) (2015) *Resuscitation Guidelines*. https://www.resus.org.uk/resuscitation-guidelines (accessed March 2018).

Resnick R (1980) Management of shoulder dystocia girdle. *Clin Obstet Gynecol* 23: 559–64.

Rey E, Boulet LP (2007) Asthma in pregnancy. *BMJ* 334: 582–5.

Roberts I, Shakur H, Afolabi A, Brohi K, Coats T, Dewan Y; CRASH-2 Collaborators (2011) The importance of early treatment with tranexamic acid in bleeding trauma patients: an exploratory analysis of the CRASH-2 randomised controlled trial. *Lancet* 377(9771): 1096–101.

Rull G (2016) *Intra-abdominal Sepsis and Abscesses*. http://patient.info/doctor/Intra-abdominal-Sepsis-and-Abscesses.htm (accessed March 2018).

Uygur D, Kis S, Tuncer R, Ozcan FS, Erkaya S (2002) Risk factors and infant outcomes associated with umbilical cord prolapse [Abstract]. *Int J Gynaecol Obstet* 78(2): 127–30.

Woollard M, Simpson H, Hinshaw K, Wieteska S (2008) Training for prehospital obstetric emergencies. *Emerg Med J* 25(7): 392–3.

Woollard M, Todd I (2006) Legal issues. In: Greaves I, Porter K, Hodgetts T, Woollard M (eds) *Emergency Care: A textbook for paramedics*, 2nd edn. Edinburgh: Saunders Elsevier.

Further reading

Birthrights (2015) *Unassisted Birth: The legal position (factsheet)*. http://www.birthrights.org.uk/library/factsheets/Unassisted-Birth.pdf (accessed March 2018).

Burke CS, Salas E, Wilson-Donnelly K, Priest H (2004) How to turn a team of experts into an expert medical team: guidance from the aviation and military communities. *Qual Saf Health Care* 13 (Suppl 1): i96–i104.

Data Protection (Amendment) Act 2003. London: HMSO.

Deakin C, Brown S, Jewkes F, Lockey D, Lyon R, Moore F, Perkins G, Whitbread M (2015) *UK Resuscitation Guidelines 2015: Prehospital Resuscitation*. London: UK Resuscitation Council. https://www.resus.org.uk/resuscitation-guidelines/prehospital-resuscitation (accessed March 2018).

DoH (Department of Health) (2005) *Mental Capacity Act*. London, HMSO.

Endsley MR (1995) Toward a theory of situation awareness in dynamic systems. *Human Factors* 37(1): 32–64.

HSCIC (Health and Social Care Information Centre) (2015) *NHS Maternity Statistics – England, 2013–14*. NHS Digital. http://www.hscic.gov.uk/catalogue/PUB16725/nhs-mate-eng-2013-14-summ-repo-rep.pdf (accessed March 2018).

Jo's Cervical Cancer Trust (2017) *Large Loop Excision of Transformation Zone*. https://www.jostrust.org.uk/about-cervical-cancer/cervical-cancer/treatments/surgery/lletz (accessed March 2018).

Leonard M, Graham S, Bonacum D (2004) The human factor: the critical importance of effective teamwork and communication in providing safe care. *Qual Saf Health Care* 13 (Suppl 1): i85–i90.

MBRRACE-UK. *Mothers and Babies: Reducing risk through audits and confidential enquiries across the UK*. https://www.npeu.ox.ac.uk/mbrrace-uk (accessed March 2018).

McQueen A (2011) Ectopic pregnancy: risk factors, diagnostic procedures and treatment. *Nursing Standard* 25(37): 49–56.

Murphy VE, Clifton VL, Gibson PG (2006) Asthma exacerbations during pregnance: incidence and association with adverse pregnancy outcomes. *Thorax* 61: 169–76.

NHS Choices (2014) *Colposcopy – Treatments*. http://www.nhs.uk/Conditions/Colposcopy/Pages/Treatment.aspx (accessed March 2018).

NHS Choices (2015) *Pelvic Organ Prolapse – Treatment*. http://www.nhs.uk/Conditions/Prolapse-of-the-uterus/Pages/Treatment.aspx (accessed March 2018).

NICE (National Institute for Health and Care Excellence) (2008) *Antenatal Care*. NICE Clinical Guideline 62 (updated 2010). Manchester: NICE.

NICE (National Institute for Health and Care Excellence) (2010) *Venous Thromboembolism: Reducing the risk for patients in hospital*. NICE Clinical Guideline 92. London: NICE.

Pre-Obstetric Emergency Training: A Practical Approach, Second Edition. Edited by Mark Woolcock.
© 2019 John Wiley & Sons Ltd. Published 2019 by John Wiley & Sons Ltd.

NICE (National Institute for Care Excellence) (2014) *Intrapartum Care for Healthy Women and Babies*. NICE Clinical Guideline (CG190). NICE London.

NICE (National Institute for Health and Care Excellence) (2015) *Mastitis and Breast Abscess*. cks.nice.org.uk/mastitis-and-breast-abscess (accessed March 2018).

NICE (National Institute for Health and Care Excellence) (2015) *Planning Place of Birth Antenatal Care Pathway*. http://pathways.nice.org.uk/pathways/antenatal-care-for-uncomplicated-pregnancies/antenatal-care-for-uncomplicated-pregancies-planning-place-of-birth (accessed March 2018).

NQB (National Quality Board) (2013) *Human Factors in Healthcare: A concordat from the National Quality Board*. http://www.england.nhs.uk/wp-content/uploads/2013/11/nqb-hum-fact-concord.pdf (accessed March 2018).

Perinatal Institute for Maternal and Child Health (2015) *Pregnancy Notes: About the notes*. http://www.preg.info/PregnancyNotes/Default.aspx (accessed March 2018).

Plous S (1993) *The Psychology of Judgment and Decision Making*. New York: McGraw-Hill.

RCOG (Royal College of Obstetricians and Gynaecologists) (2015) *Birth After Previous Caesarean Birth*. Green-top Guideline No. 45. London: RCOG.

RCPSG (Royal College of Physicians and Surgeons of Glasgow). *Maternal Health*. https://rcpsg.ac.uk/college/influencing-healthcare/policy/maternal-health (accessed March 2018).

Reason J (1997) *Managing the Risks of Organisational Accidents*. Aldershot: Ashgate Publishing.

Reason J (2010) *The Human Contribution: Unsafe acts, accidents and heroic recoveries*. Farnham: Ashgate Publishing.

Salas E, Burke CS, Stagal KC (2004) Developing teams and team leaders: strategies and principles. In: Day D, Zaccaro S, Haplin SM (eds) *Leader Development for Transforming Organisations. Growing leaders for tomorrow*. Mahwah, NJ: Lawrence-Erlbaum, pp. 325–58.

Singer, M, Deutschman C, Warren-Seymour MD (2016) The Third International Consensus definition for sepsis and septic shock. *JAMA* 315(8): 801–10.

Surviving Sepsis Campaign (2012) International Guidelines for Management of Severe Sepsis and Septic Schock: 2012. http://www.sccm.org/Documents/SSC-Guidelines.pdf (accessed March 2018).

Tyler S (2012) *Commissioning Maternity Services: A resource pack to support clinical commissioning groups*. London: NHS Commissioning Board.

Vincent C, Neale G, Woloshynowych M (2001) Adverse events in British hospitals: preliminary retrospective record review. *BMJ* 322: 517–19.

WHO, UNICEF, UNFPA, World Bank Group and the United Nations Population Division. *Maternal Mortality Ratio (modelled estimate, per 100,000 live births)*. http://data.worldbank.org/indicator/SH.STA.MMRT (accessed March 2018).

Index

Note: Italicised *b*, *f* and *t* refer to numbered boxes, figures and tables